COMFORT FOODS FOR CHRONIC KIDNEY DISEASE

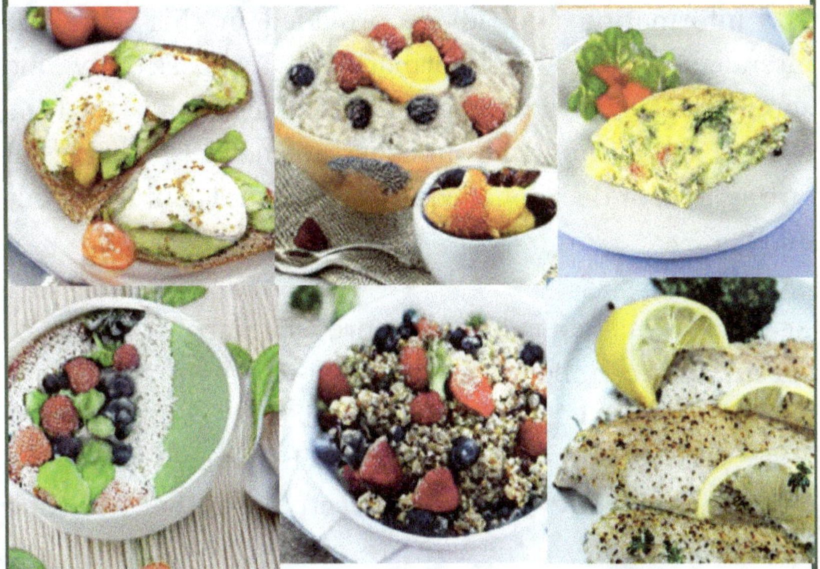

NOURISHING, KIDNEY-FRIENDLY RECIPES TO ENJOY WHILE MANAGING DIALYSIS, MINERALS, AND NUTRITION

ADELINE GREEN

Disclaimer

The information and advice provided in this work are intended for general informational purposes only and should not be considered as professional, medical, or legal advice. The author and publisher are not responsible for any actions or decisions made based on the content of this book.

Readers should consult with appropriate professionals for specific advice tailored to their individual situations. The author and publisher disclaim any liability for any loss or risk, personal or otherwise, which is incurred as a consequence, directly or indirectly, of the use and application of any of the contents of this book.

While every effort has been made to ensure the accuracy and completeness of the information in this publication, the author and publisher assume no responsibility for errors, inaccuracies, or omissions, or any loss or damage arising from the display or use of this information.

Table of Contents

Introduction

Do you ever find yourself yearning for the warmth and familiarity of comfort foods, only to be held back by the challenges of managing Chronic Kidney Disease (CKD)? If so, you're not alone. The journey of navigating kidney health can often feel like a daunting road, filled with dietary restrictions and the constant need to balance dialysis, minerals, and nutrition. But fear not, for within the pages of this book lies a beacon of hope and nourishment. "Comfort Foods for Chronic Kidney Disease: Nourishing, Kidney-Friendly Recipes to Enjoy While Managing Dialysis, Minerals, and Nutrition."

In a world where every bite matters, this book is not just a collection of recipes; it's a companion for those facing the daily challenges of CKD. We understand the emotional toll that restrictive diets can take, and that's why we've curated a selection of comforting, soul-soothing recipes designed to bring joy and satisfaction back to your dining experience.

The Challenge and The Solution:

Living with Chronic Kidney Disease is a journey that demands constant attention to what you eat. The challenge lies in finding a balance between nourishing your body and adhering to the dietary restrictions that come with managing CKD. It's a path often paved with questions, "What can I eat? How do I ensure my meals are kidney-friendly?" Craving the comfort of your favorite foods without compromising your kidneys?

This book is your culinary compass, navigating you through delicious recipes, dialysis management, and essential mineral know-how to empower your nutritional journey.

Benefits of the Book:

Flavorful Liberation: Say goodbye to bland and monotonous meals. Discover a world where kidney-friendly can also mean palate-pleasing. From hearty breakfasts to indulgent desserts, each recipe is crafted to satisfy both your taste buds and your nutritional needs.

Empowerment Through Knowledge: Knowledge is power, especially when it comes to managing your health. Unravel the mysteries of CKD, gain insights into dialysis, minerals, and nutrition, and empower yourself with the tools to make informed, health-conscious choices.

Emotional Well-being: We understand that food is not just fuel; it's a source of joy, comfort, and connection. By embracing the recipes in this book, you're not just nourishing your body, you're feeding your soul, finding comfort in each carefully crafted dish.

Embark on a culinary journey that transcends the limitations of a kidney-friendly diet. "Comfort Foods for Chronic Kidney Disease" is not just a book; it's an invitation to rediscover the pleasure of eating, to find solace in flavors, and to savor every bite on the path to better kidney health. It's time to turn the page on dietary restrictions and embrace a world where comfort and kidney care coexist harmoniously. Your journey to delicious well-being begins now.

Chapter 1
Managing Dialysis

Overview of Dialysis

In the tapestry of life, our health often takes center stage, weaving its threads through the daily tapestry of our existence. For those facing the challenges of Chronic Kidney Disease, this journey can be particularly intricate, with the delicate dance of managing dialysis playing a crucial role. As we delve into the first chapter of "Comfort Foods for Chronic Kidney Disease," let us embark on a narrative that brings understanding and empathy to the forefront.

Sarah's Story: A Journey of Resilience

Meet Sarah, a spirited soul who found herself navigating the uncharted waters of dialysis. Her story is not just hers but resonates with countless individuals facing the same path. Sarah's initial encounter with dialysis was akin to stepping into the unknown. The whirring machines, the sterile environment, it all felt overwhelming. But within those clinical confines, she discovered a community, a network of individuals sharing similar fears, hopes, and, most importantly, a resilience that sparked a kinship among them.

Dialysis is not merely a medical procedure; it's a chapter in the lives of many, a shared experience that transcends the confines of a treatment room. It's about the quiet courage to face the unknown, the strength required to adapt, and the resilience to keep moving forward.

Within these pages, we approach the topic of dialysis not as a clinical process but as a shared experience. The intention is not to overwhelm with medical jargon but to offer a compassionate understanding. We acknowledge the emotional weight that accompanies the hum of the dialysis machine, the vulnerability felt in the presence of healthcare providers, and the resilience required to sustain this journey.

Managing dialysis is not just about physical well-being; it's a testament to emotional strength. As you read through this chapter, envision it as a conversation with a friend, a guide through the labyrinth of dialysis where warmth and understanding prevail. Let these words serve as a beacon, illuminating the path with empathy and compassion.

To those navigating the currents of dialysis, this chapter extends a warm embrace. You are not alone in this journey. Sarah's story, and the stories yet to unfold, remind us that within the challenges of dialysis lies a tapestry of strength, resilience, and shared humanity. As we explore the overview of dialysis, let it be a reminder that this chapter is not just about managing a medical procedure; it's about managing life with grace and fortitude.

So, come, let us embark on this chapter together with empathy in our hearts, understanding in our minds, and the shared warmth of connection.

Dietary Guidelines for Dialysis Patients

Navigating the waters of Chronic Kidney Disease requires a delicate dance, especially for those undergoing dialysis. As we venture into the realm of dietary guidelines, envision it as a roadmap designed to empower and nourish. Beyond the clinical recommendations, these guidelines are crafted with the understanding that every meal is an opportunity for healing, resilience, and well-being.

Understanding the Basics:

Before we dive deep, let's establish a foundation. Dialysis, a vital component in managing kidney health, brings about unique dietary considerations. The aim is twofold: to provide the necessary nutrients for overall health and to manage the levels of substances that the kidneys would typically filter out, such as potassium, phosphorus, and sodium.

Balancing Nutrients:

1. Protein: Dialysis can alter protein needs. Sufficient protein intake is crucial for preserving muscle tissue and general well-being. However, the type and amount of protein may need adjustment to prevent waste buildup.

2. Fluid Intake: Dialysis affects the body's fluid balance. Monitoring fluid intake is crucial to prevent fluid overload, which can strain the heart. Delight in hydrating foods and regulate fluid intake with precision.

Watchful Eye on Minerals:

1. Potassium: With impaired kidney function, potassium levels can rise. Opt for low-potassium fruits and vegetables, and manage portion sizes to keep levels in check.

2. Phosphorus: A diligent approach to phosphorus is vital, as it can accumulate in the blood. Choose low-phosphorus foods and consider phosphorus binders as recommended.

3. Sodium: Dialysis doesn't eliminate sodium as effectively as healthy kidneys. Limiting sodium helps control blood pressure and fluid balance. Embrace herbs and spices for flavor, minimizing reliance on salt.

Creating Kidney-Friendly Meals:

1. Diverse Fruits and Vegetables: Explore a rainbow of fruits and vegetables, selecting those lower in potassium and phosphorus. Enjoy a variety to ensure a spectrum of nutrients.

2. Quality Protein Sources: Opt for high-quality protein from lean meats, poultry, fish, eggs, and dairy. Adjust protein intake based on individual needs and dialysis type.

3. Whole Grains and Legumes: Embrace the wholesome goodness of whole grains and legumes, balancing fiber intake. Choose varieties lower in phosphorus.

Personalization and Monitoring:

Dialysis patients are unique, and dietary guidelines should reflect individual health, preferences, and treatment plans. Regular monitoring of blood work and collaboration with healthcare providers ensure ongoing adjustments for optimal well-being.

A Culinary Journey of Healing:

In this chapter, dietary guidelines are not restrictions but opportunities for culinary creativity. Each meal is a canvas, allowing you to craft dishes that align with kidney health without compromising flavor. Embrace the art of nourishing your body, savoring each bite as a step toward holistic well-being.

Let these guidelines be a companion on your journey, offering clarity, empowerment, and a newfound appreciation for the intersection of health and flavor. As you embrace the art of mindful eating, remember that each meal is a celebration of resilience and a step towards a healthier, vibrant life.

Recipes to Support Dialysis

Recipe 1. Vegetable and Chicken Stir-Fry

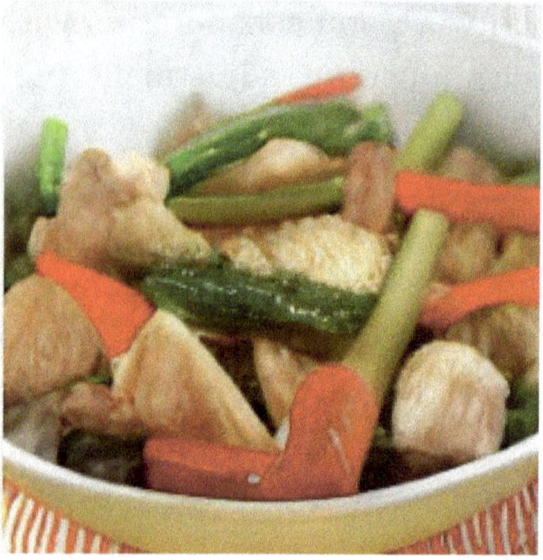

Ingredients:

- Boneless, skinless chicken breasts, sliced
- Assorted vegetables (bell peppers, zucchini, carrots), sliced
- Low-sodium soy sauce
- Garlic (minced)
- Ginger (grated)
- Olive oil
- Brown rice or quinoa (cooked)

Preparation:

1. In a wok or skillet, heat olive oil over medium-high heat.
2. Add sliced chicken and cook until browned and fully cooked.
3. Add minced garlic and grated ginger, stir for a minute.
4. Add sliced vegetables and cook until they are tender-crisp.
5. Drizzle low-sodium soy sauce over the mixture, stir to combine.
6. Serve over a bed of cooked brown rice or quinoa.

Recipe 2. Baked Lemon Herb Tilapia

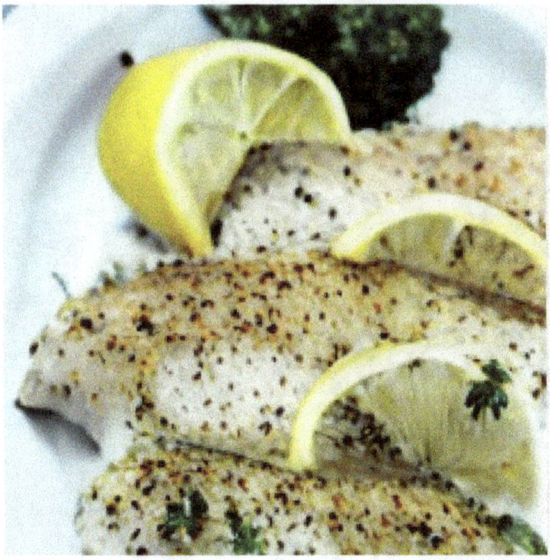

Ingredients:

- Tilapia fillets
- Lemon juice
- Aromatic herbs, including parsley, dill, and thyme, finely minced.
- Olive oil
- Garlic (minced)
- Salt and pepper to taste

Preparation:

1. Preheat the oven to 375°F (190°C).
2. Place tilapia fillets in a baking dish.
3. In a small bowl, mix lemon juice, chopped herbs, olive oil, minced garlic, salt, and pepper.
4. Pour the mixture over the tilapia fillets, ensuring they are well-coated.
5. Bake for 15-20 minutes or until the fish flakes easily with a fork.
6. Serve with steamed green beans or a side of your choice.

Recipe 3. Quinoa and Black Bean Salad

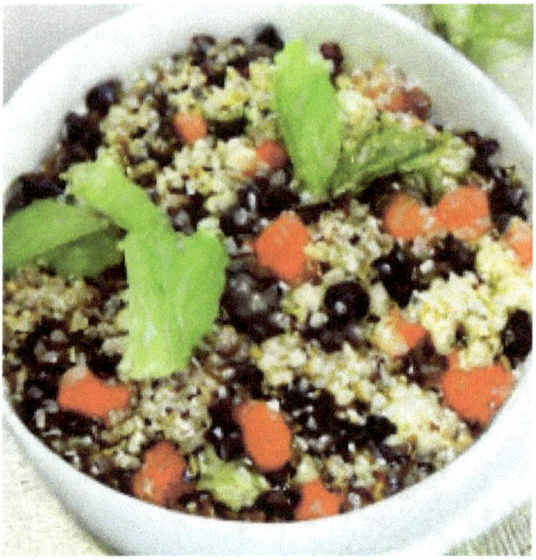

Ingredients:

- Cooked quinoa
- Black beans (canned, rinsed and drained)
- Corn kernels (fresh or frozen)
- Cherry tomatoes, halved
- Red onion, finely chopped
- Cilantro, chopped
- Lime juice
- Olive oil

Salt and pepper to taste

Preparation:

1. In a large bowl, combine cooked quinoa, black beans, corn, cherry tomatoes, red onion, and cilantro.
2. In a small bowl, whisk together lime juice, olive oil, salt, and pepper.
3. Drizzle the vinaigrette over the leafy greens, ensuring even distribution, and then gently fold to integrate the flavors.
4. Refrigerate for at least 30 minutes before serving to let the flavors meld.

Chapter 2
Essential Minerals for Kidney Health

Role of Minerals in Kidney Function

In the intricate dance of physiology, minerals play the role of unsung heroes, quietly orchestrating vital functions within the human body. As we embark on Chapter 2 of "Comfort Foods for Chronic Kidney Disease," let us unravel the tapestry of essential minerals and their profound impact on kidney health.

Understanding the Symphony: The Role of Minerals in Kidney Function

The kidneys, those remarkable organs nestled within our lower backs, are not mere filters; they are conductors of a symphony of mineral balance. Imagine them as skilled maestros, finely tuning the delicate interplay of minerals to maintain equilibrium. Let's explore the key minerals that harmonize within this intricate composition:

1. Sodium: The conductor's baton, sodium orchestrates fluid balance. Its measured presence ensures an optimal environment for the kidneys to function effectively, maintaining blood pressure and fluid levels.

2. Potassium: The tenor of the mineral ensemble, potassium, plays a crucial role in nerve and muscle function. In kidney health, it requires careful moderation to prevent imbalances that may arise during impaired kidney function.

3. Phosphorus: The bass notes, phosphorus, contribute to bone health and energy metabolism. Yet, in the realm of kidney health, maintaining phosphorus balance becomes a nuanced dance to prevent its accumulation in the bloodstream.

4. Calcium: A delicate pianissimo, calcium partners with phosphorus for bone health. The kidneys, in their symphonic role, manage calcium excretion and absorption to sustain this delicate balance.

5. Magnesium: The subtle percussion, magnesium, supports muscle and nerve function. Kidneys contribute to magnesium equilibrium, ensuring its presence in harmony with other minerals.

6. Chloride: Like the background hum, chloride aids in fluid balance and digestion. The kidneys fine-tune chloride levels, maintaining the delicate equilibrium crucial for overall health.

The Intricate Ballet of Mineral Balance:

In a healthy symphony, minerals move in seamless coordination. However, the melody may falter when kidneys face challenges. Chronic Kidney Disease introduces a unique cadence, requiring a nuanced approach to mineral management.

Harmonizing Mineral Intake:

1. Mindful Sodium Consumption: Moderation is the key to sodium's harmonious contribution. Embrace the flavors of herbs and spices while minimizing processed foods to maintain balance.

2. Balancing Potassium-Rich Foods: Revel in a variety of fruits and vegetables, mindful of potassium content. Individual tolerance varies, and adjustments ensure a personalized balance.

3. Phosphorus Awareness: Navigate the landscape of phosphorus by selecting low-phosphorus foods and considering phosphorus binders as recommended. Balancing intake is crucial to prevent complications.

Cultivating Harmony in Kidney Health:

As we explore the symphony of essential minerals, let it be a reminder that kidney health is a delicate dance. It involves not just the biological functions of the kidneys but also an awareness of the dietary choices that contribute to mineral harmony.

Within the pages of this chapter, envision a journey of understanding, where minerals are not just elements but integral notes in the melody of well-being. Let the role of minerals in kidney function resonate as a call to embrace a balanced, mindful approach to nutrition, enriching the symphony of your health.

Balancing Minerals in Your Diet

Embarking on a journey toward kidney health involves not just understanding the role of minerals but mastering the art of balance. In this chapter, we navigate the delicate terrain of "Balancing Minerals in Your Diet," treating each mineral as a note in the melody of well-being. The goal is not restriction, but rather a symphony of moderation and mindful choices.

Understanding Individual Needs:

The first step in this culinary odyssey is recognizing that each person is unique. Your mineral requirements are influenced by factors such as age, gender, overall health, and the specific challenges your kidneys face. Hence, the pursuit of balance is a personalized journey, one that considers individual needs and tolerances.

Sodium: The Flavorful Moderation

Sodium, often associated with the savory symphony of flavors, requires a delicate touch. While it adds zest to our dishes, excessive sodium can disrupt the balance and strain the kidneys. Explore the world of herbs, spices, and low-sodium alternatives to enhance flavors without compromising health.

Potassium: The Art of Variety

Potassium, abundant in fruits and vegetables, is a vital nutrient for nerve and muscle function. Embrace the rich palette of produce, but maintain a mindful variety. Balancing high-potassium and low-potassium choices ensures a diverse nutrient intake without overwhelming your kidneys.

Phosphorus: A Delicate Dance

Phosphorus, the silent partner in bone health, demands a nuanced dance in kidney care. Opt for low-phosphorus alternatives while savoring a spectrum of whole foods. Navigating phosphorus content with awareness helps maintain equilibrium without sacrificing culinary pleasure.

Calcium: A Symphony of Absorption

Calcium, the backbone of bone health, partners with phosphorus in a delicate ballet. Balance the intake of dairy and non-dairy sources, mindful of both calcium and phosphorus levels. The goal is to foster absorption while preventing imbalances that can challenge kidney function.

Magnesium: Orchestrating Nerve Function

Magnesium, often overlooked but essential, supports nerve and muscle function. While its presence is crucial, achieving balance involves incorporating magnesium-rich foods without overwhelming the delicate harmony of minerals in your diet.

Chloride: The Subtle Support

Chloride, a subtle contributor to fluid balance and digestion, plays a supporting role. Let chloride-rich foods complement your meals, providing a nuanced note in the orchestration of mineral equilibrium.

Navigating Your Culinary Symphony:

As you embark on the culinary journey of balancing minerals, think of it as a symphony, each mineral playing its part in the overall composition. Embrace variety, savor the nuances of flavors, and celebrate the art of mindful eating. Remember, this is not a rigid regimen; it's an exploration of how the symphony of minerals can coexist harmoniously within your diet.

Practical Tips for Balance:

1. Educate Yourself: Learn about the mineral content of foods and make informed choices.

2. Portion Control: Moderation is key. Control portion sizes to maintain balance.

3. Consult Your Healthcare Team: Work closely with your healthcare providers to tailor dietary choices to your specific needs.

Balancing minerals is not a chore; it's an invitation to discover the richness of a well-balanced, kidney-friendly diet. As you explore the world of flavors and nutrients, let this chapter be your guide, a companion on your journey to maintaining a harmonious symphony of health and well-being.

Mineral-Rich Recipes

Recipe 1. Lemon-herb grilled Salmon

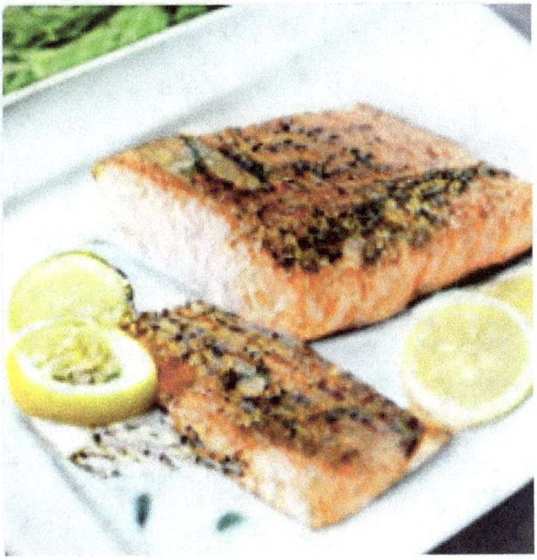

Ingredients:

- Fresh salmon fillets
- Lemon zest and juice
- Fresh herbs (such as dill, parsley, or thyme)
- Olive oil
- Garlic (minced)
- Salt and pepper to taste

Preparation:

1. Marinate salmon in a mixture of lemon zest, lemon juice, herbs, olive oil, minced garlic, salt, and pepper.
2. Grill until salmon is flaky and infused with the citrusy herb goodness.
3. This recipe not only provides high-quality protein but also offers a dose of heart-healthy omega-3 fatty acids.

Recipe 2. Quinoa and Vegetable Stir-Fry

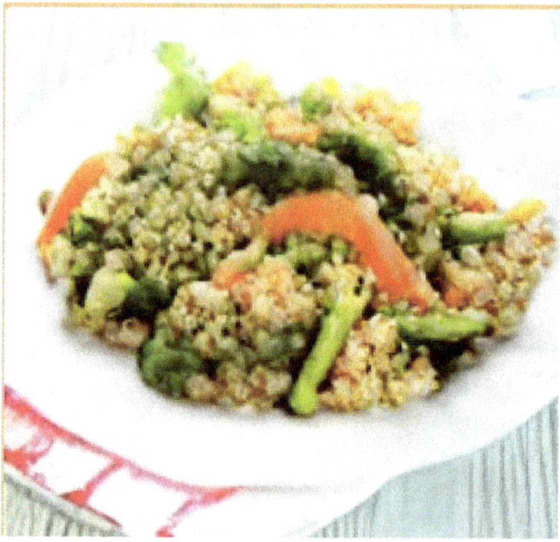

Ingredients:

- Quinoa
- Assorted vegetables (bell peppers, broccoli, carrots)
- Low-sodium soy sauce
- Garlic (minced)
- Ginger (grated)
- Sesame oil
- Scallions (chopped)

Preparation:

1. Cook quinoa and set aside.
2. Stir-fry a colorful medley of vegetables in a wok with garlic, ginger, and a splash of low-sodium soy sauce.
3. Toss in the cooked quinoa, drizzle with sesame oil, and garnish with chopped scallions.
4. This nutrient-packed dish is rich in fiber, essential minerals, and a spectrum of vitamins.

Recipe 4. Spinach and Chickpea Salad

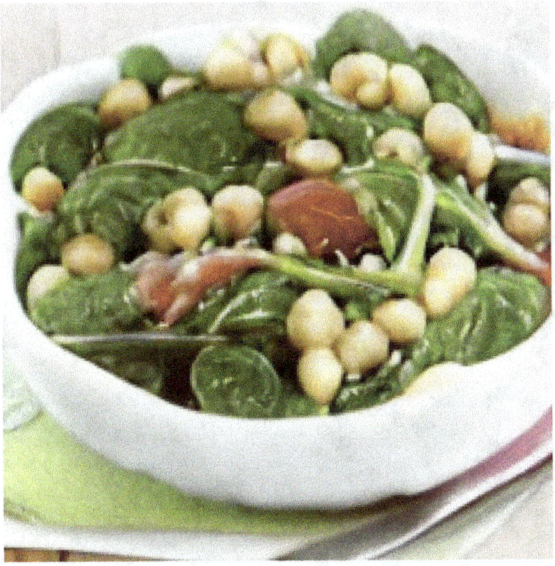

Ingredients:

- Fresh spinach leaves
- Chickpeas (cooked)
- Cherry tomatoes (halved)
- Feta cheese (crumbled)
- Olive oil
- Balsamic vinegar
- Dried oregano
- Salt and pepper to taste

Preparation:

1. Layer Greek yogurt with Toss together fresh spinach, chickpeas, cherry tomatoes, and crumbled feta cheese.
2. Dress the salad with a simple vinaigrette made with olive oil, balsamic vinegar, dried oregano, salt, and pepper.
3. This salad is a mineral-rich delight, offering iron from spinach, protein from chickpeas, and the savory goodness of feta.

Recipe 5. Sweet Potato and Kale Hash

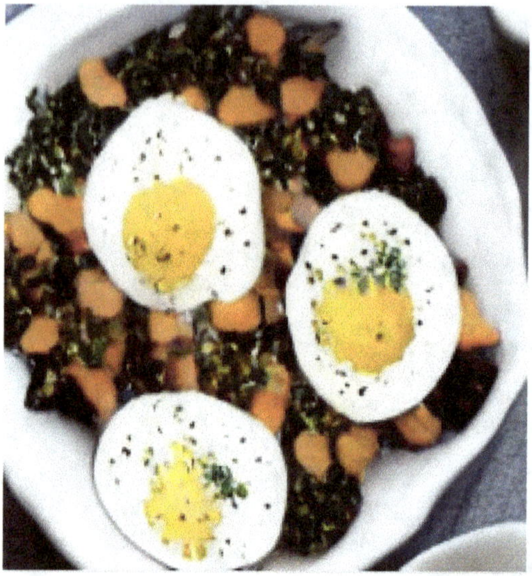

Ingredients:

- Sweet potatoes (diced)
- Kale (chopped)
- Red onion (sliced)
- Garlic (minced)
- Olive oil
- Paprika

Salt and pepper to taste

Preparation:

1. Sauté diced sweet potatoes, chopped kale, and sliced red onion in olive oil with minced garlic, paprika, salt, and pepper.
2. This nutrient-dense hash is loaded with potassium, vitamins, and antioxidants from sweet potatoes and kale..

Chapter 3
Nutrition for Kidney Health

Nutritional Needs for Chronic Kidney Disease

In the canvas of health, nutrition forms the vibrant strokes that contribute to the masterpiece of well-being. As we delve into the heart of "Comfort Foods for Chronic Kidney Disease," Chapter 3 invites us to explore the intricate tapestry of nutritional needs specific to those navigating the path of Chronic Kidney Disease (CKD). This chapter is not merely a guide; it's a culinary journey towards holistic health.

Unveiling the Mosaic: Nutritional Needs for Chronic Kidney Disease

Understanding the nutritional landscape of CKD requires a blend of science and artistry. It's about harmonizing nutrients to support kidney function while maintaining overall health. Let's unveil the mosaic of nutritional needs, recognizing that each nutrient is a vital hue contributing to the vibrancy of well-being.

Protein: A Balancing Act

Protein, the cornerstone of vitality, takes center stage in the CKD nutritional narrative. While essential for muscle maintenance and overall health, managing protein intake becomes a delicate balancing act. This chapter guides you through the intricacies, helping you strike the perfect balance to support your body without overburdening your kidneys.

Calories: Nourishing the Body and Soul

Calories, the energy currency of life, play a pivotal role in CKD nutrition. Balancing calorie intake is not just about numbers; it's about nourishing the body and soul. Discover how to meet your energy needs while embracing a variety of nutrient-dense, kidney-friendly foods.

Fiber: Embracing Digestive Harmony

Fiber, often an unsung hero, contributes to digestive health and overall well-being. This chapter explores the art of embracing fiber without compromising on dietary restrictions. Discover a world of fiber-rich foods that bring both digestive harmony and nutritional support.

Fluids: Sipping Sustainably

Fluid intake is a dance between hydration and moderation in CKD. Explore the nuances of fluid management, recognizing the importance of staying hydrated while being mindful of restrictions. Learn how to savor the goodness of hydrating foods and manage fluids without sacrificing taste.

Vitamins and Minerals: Nurturing Nutrient Balance

Beyond the macronutrients, the world of vitamins and minerals is a garden of essential nutrients. This chapter guides you through the nutritional landscape, helping you cultivate a balance of vitamins and minerals to support overall health and kidney function.

Tailoring Nutrition to Your Journey:

The beauty of nutritional needs for CKD lies in its adaptability. This chapter encourages you to view nutrition not as a set of restrictions but as a flexible framework. Tailor your dietary choices to your unique journey, embracing the abundance of flavors and nutrients that contribute to your well-being.

Navigating the Culinary Seas:

As you navigate the culinary seas of CKD nutrition, envision it as a voyage of discovery. Each nutrient is not just a component; it's a brushstroke adding depth to the canvas of your health. Let this chapter be your compass, guiding you through the nutritional needs of CKD with wisdom, practical insights, and a celebration of the nourishing power of food.

Creating a Well-Balanced Diet

In the culinary journey of managing Chronic Kidney Disease (CKD), creating a well-balanced diet is akin to composing a symphony - each nutrient, flavor, and texture playing a crucial role in the harmony of well-being. Chapter 3 has acquainted us with the nutritional needs specific to CKD, and now, we embark on the art of crafting a well-balanced diet tailored to support kidney health.

Harmony in Macronutrients: The Protein Puzzle

Balancing Act with Protein:

Protein, a vital player in the nutritional orchestra, demands a balancing act for those with CKD. While essential for muscle maintenance and overall health, it's about quality over quantity. Lean towards high-quality sources like poultry, fish, and plant-based proteins, and tailor your intake to meet individual needs without overburdening your kidneys.

Melody of Micronutrients: A Rainbow of Nutrients

Vitamins and Minerals:

In crafting a well-balanced diet, the spotlight also shines on the symphony of vitamins and minerals. Ensure your plate is adorned with a variety of colorful fruits and vegetables, each offering a unique blend of essential nutrients. Embrace the rainbow, and let the hues of your meals reflect the diversity of vitamins and minerals crucial for kidney health.

Rhythm of Fiber: Nurturing Digestive Well-being

Embracing Fiber:

Fiber, the rhythm section of the nutritional ensemble, is often underestimated. Its role in supporting digestive health is paramount for individuals with CKD. Incorporate fiber-rich foods like whole grains, fruits, and vegetables, ensuring a melody that resonates with both nourishment and digestive harmony.

Fluids: A Hydration Sonata

Sipping Sustainably:

Fluid management in CKD is a delicate dance, and crafting a well-balanced diet involves a hydration sonata. Sip sustainably by incorporating hydrating foods and being mindful of fluid restrictions. Let your beverage choices contribute to both the melody of hydration and the health of your kidneys.

Variety: A Symphony of Flavors and Textures

Diverse Flavors and Textures:

Variety is the spice of life, and crafting a well-balanced diet, adds the zest to your culinary symphony. Explore diverse flavors and textures, incorporating a spectrum of foods while adhering to kidney-friendly guidelines. Let your meals be a celebration of taste, ensuring both satisfaction and nutritional support.

Personalization: Your Unique Musical Composition

Tailoring to Your Journey:

No two musical compositions are identical, and similarly, no two individuals with CKD have the same dietary needs. Personalization is the key. Tailor your well-balanced diet to your unique journey, considering individual preferences, health status, and the ever-evolving nature of kidney health.

Practical Tips for Your Culinary Composition:

1. Meal Planning: Strategically plan your meals to ensure a balance of macronutrients and micronutrients.

2. Portion Control: Moderation is crucial. Control portion sizes to avoid overloading your system.

3. Consult Your Healthcare Team: Collaborate with your healthcare providers to fine-tune your diet based on regular check-ups and evolving health needs.

In the realm of CKD management, creating a well-balanced diet is not a rigid prescription but a symphony waiting to be composed. Let this chapter be your musical score, guiding you through the art of nourishing your body and soul, one well-balanced meal at a time.

Nutrient-Packed Recipes

Recipe 1. Quinoa and Vegetable Buddha Bowl

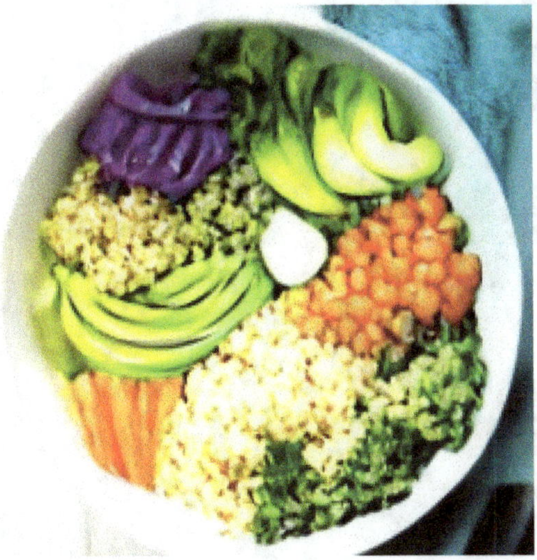

Ingredients:

- Fresh spinach leaves
- Quinoa, cooked
- Mixed vegetables (bell peppers, cherry tomatoes, broccoli)
- Avocado, sliced
- Chickpeas, roasted
- Olive oil
- Lemon juice
- Fresh herbs (cilantro, parsley)
- Salt and pepper to taste

Preparation:

1. Arrange cooked quinoa in a bowl.
2. Surround with a vibrant medley of mixed vegetables, sliced avocado, and roasted chickpeas.
3. Drizzle with olive oil and lemon juice.
4. Garnish with fresh herbs, salt, and pepper.
5. This Buddha Bowl is a nutrient-packed feast, rich in plant-based protein, fiber, and essential minerals.

Recipe 2. Salmon and Asparagus Foil Packets

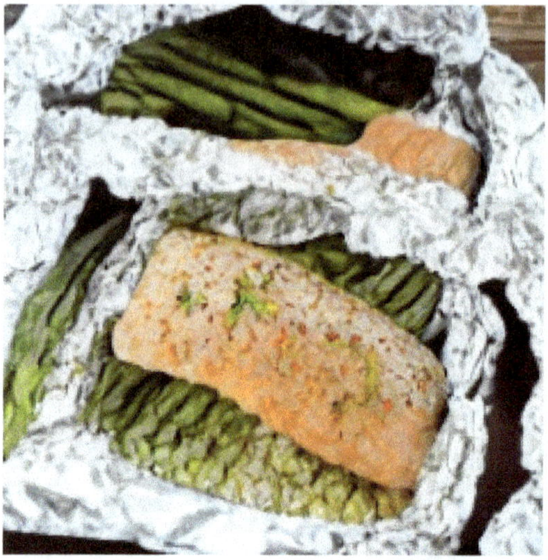

Ingredients:

- Salmon fillets
- Asparagus spears
- Lemon slices
- Garlic, minced
- Olive oil
- Fresh dill
- Salt and pepper to taste

Preparation:

1. Place salmon fillets and asparagus on a sheet of foil.
2. Top with lemon slices, minced garlic, and fresh dill.
3. Brush the salmon with olive oil and season generously with salt and pepper.
4. Securely wrap the foil packets and bake in a preheated oven at [specific temperature] until the salmon is cooked through.
5. This recipe offers omega-3 fatty acids, protein, and a burst of flavorful nutrition.

Recipe 3. Spinach and Berry Smoothie Bowl

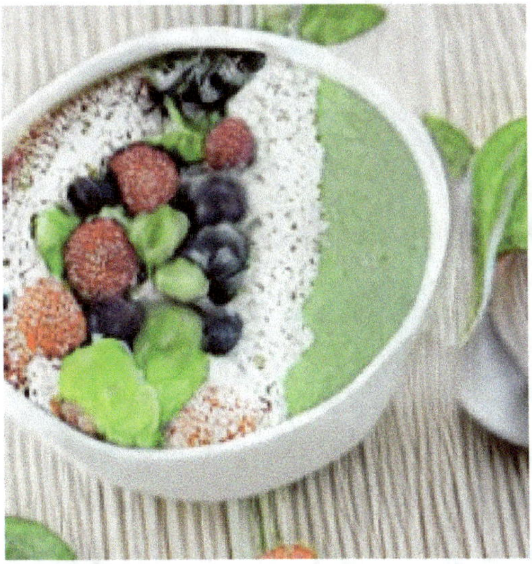

Ingredients:

- Fresh spinach
- Mixed berries (strawberries, blueberries, raspberries)
- Banana
- Greek yogurt
- Almond milk
- Chia seeds
- Granola

Preparation:

1. Blend spinach, mixed berries, banana, Greek yogurt, and almond milk until smooth.
2. Pour the smoothie into a bowl.
3. Top with chia seeds and granola for added texture.
4. This vibrant smoothie bowl is packed with antioxidants, vitamins, and fiber.

Recipe 4. Egg and Vegetable Frittata

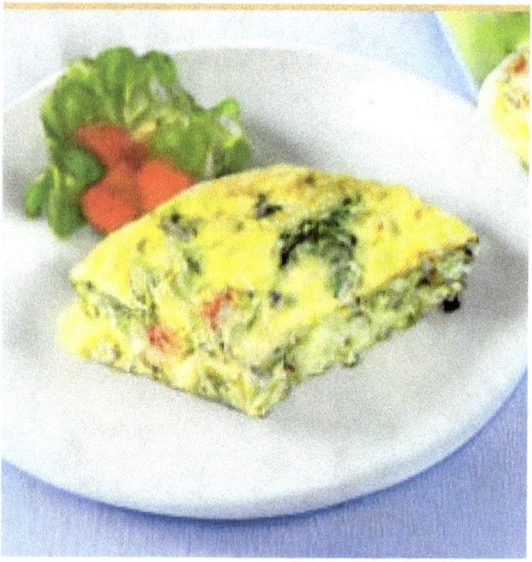

Ingredients:

- Eggs
- Bell peppers, diced
- Spinach, chopped
- Cherry tomatoes, halved
- Feta cheese, crumbled
- Olive oil
- Fresh herbs (basil, thyme)

Salt and pepper to taste

Preparation:

1. Whisk eggs in a bowl and set aside.
2. Sauté bell peppers, spinach, and cherry tomatoes in olive oil.
3. Pour the whisked eggs over the vegetables.
4. Sprinkle with feta cheese and fresh herbs. Season with salt and pepper.
5. Bake until the frittata is set and golden.
6. This protein-packed frittata is a delightful way to incorporate vegetables into your diet.

Recipe 5. Berry and Walnut Quinoa Salad

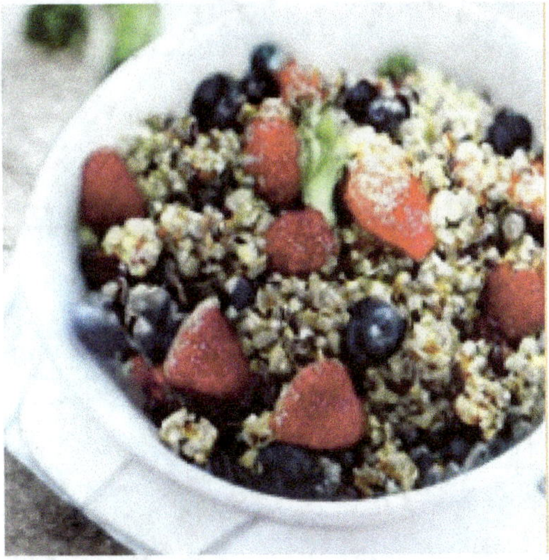

Ingredients:

- Quinoa, cooked
- Mixed berries (strawberries, blueberries, blackberries)
- Walnuts, chopped
- Feta cheese, crumbled
- Balsamic vinaigrette dressing
- Fresh mint, chopped
- Salt and pepper to taste

Preparation:

1. Combine cooked quinoa, mixed berries, chopped walnuts, and crumbled feta in a bowl.
2. Drizzle with balsamic vinaigrette dressing.
3. Garnish with fresh mint and season with salt and pepper.
4. This refreshing salad is a nutrient-packed delight with a perfect balance of sweet and savory.

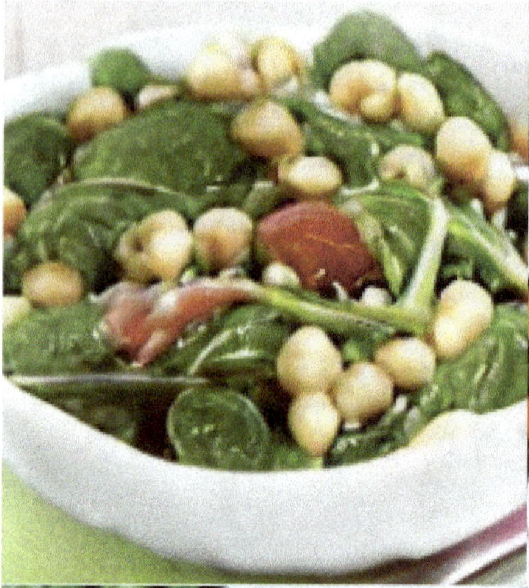
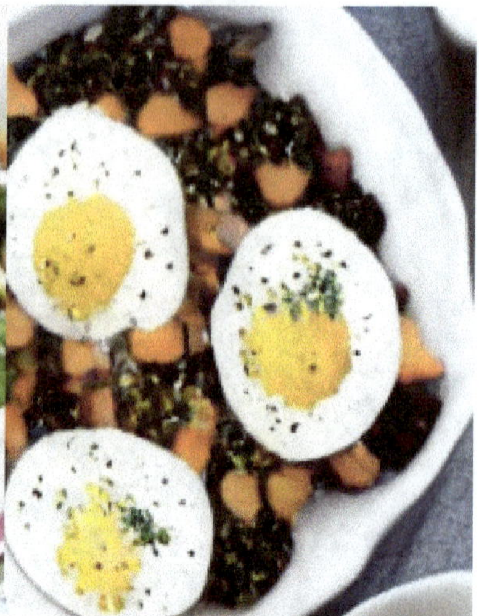
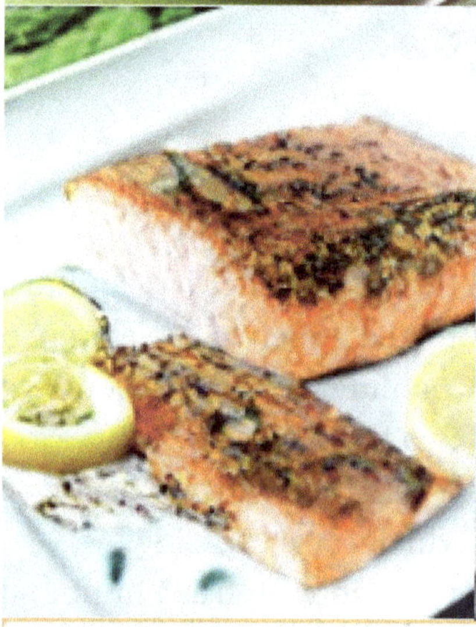
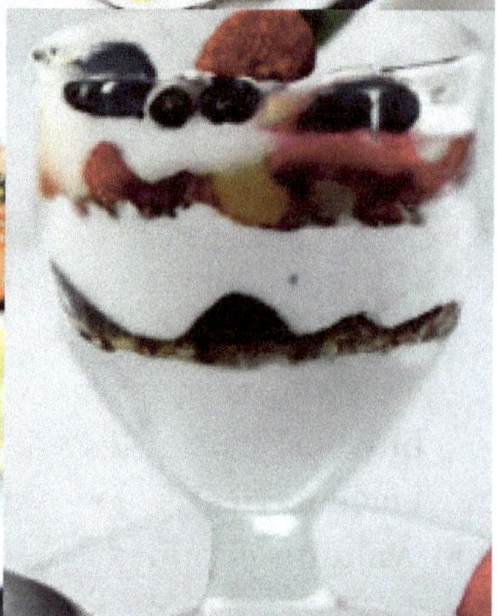
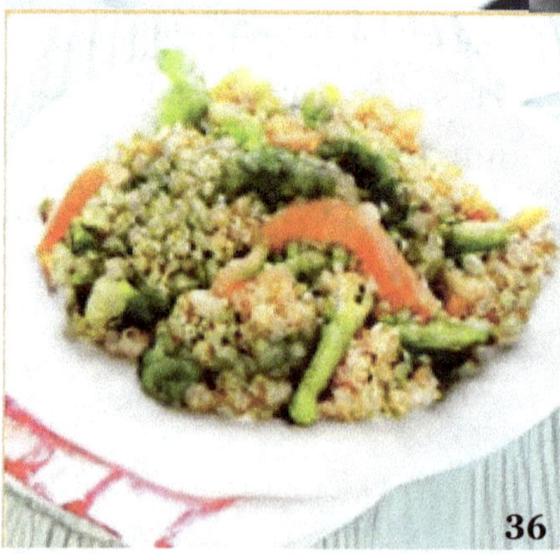
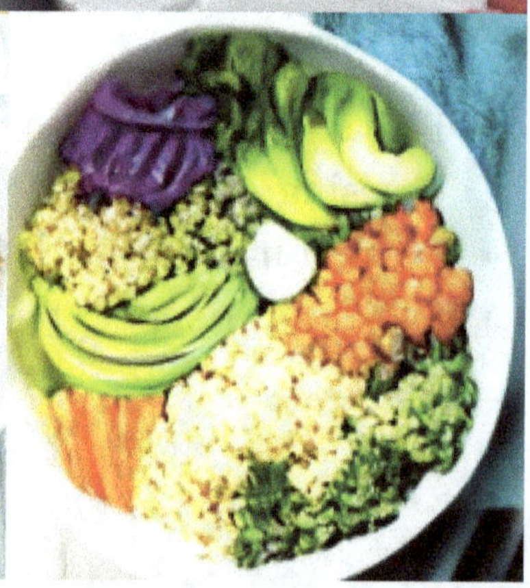

Chapter 4
Comforting Breakfasts

Hearty Morning Start

Recipe 1. Wholesome Oatmeal with Fresh Fruit Medley

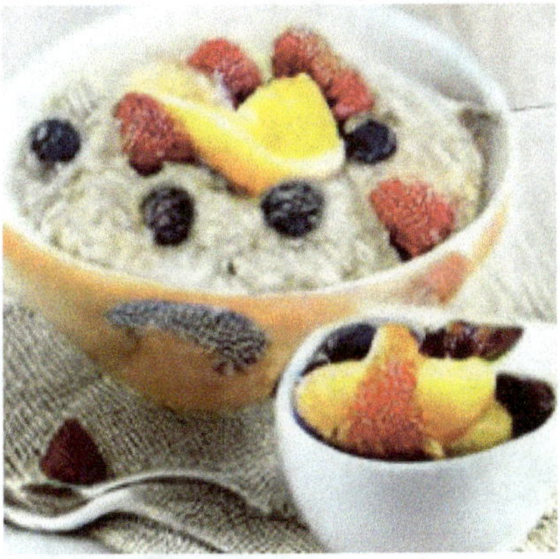

Ingredients:

- Rolled oats
- Water or low-phosphorus milk
- Mixed berries (strawberries, blueberries, raspberries)
- Banana, sliced
- Chia seeds
- Honey or maple syrup

Preparation:

1. Cook rolled oats with water or low-phosphorus milk until creamy.
2. Top with a vibrant medley of mixed berries, sliced banana, and a sprinkle of chia seeds.
3. garnish with a drizzle of honey or maple syrup for a touch of sweetness.
4. This comforting oatmeal provides a hearty dose of fiber, antioxidants, and essential vitamins.

Recipe 2. Avocado and Tomato Toast with Poached Eggs

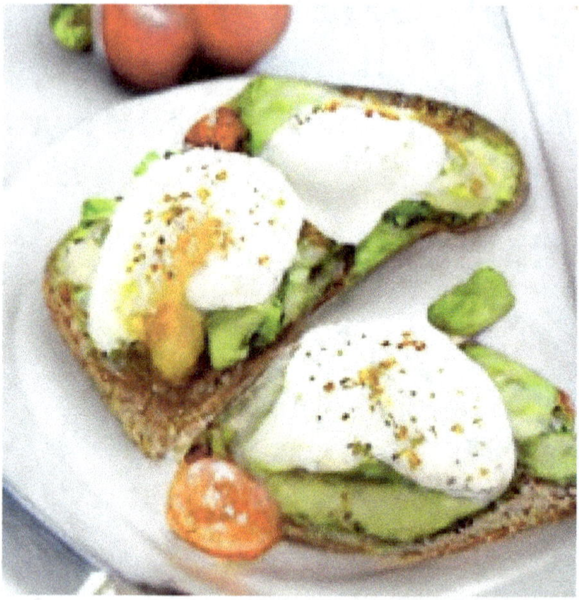

Ingredients:

- Whole-grain bread
- Ripe avocado, mashed
- Cherry tomatoes, sliced
- Eggs, poached
- Olive oil
- Salt and pepper to taste

Preparation:

1. Toast whole-grain bread and spread mashed avocado on top.
2. Arrange sliced cherry tomatoes over the avocado.
3. Top with poached eggs.
4. Garnish with a touch of olive oil and a judicious seasoning of salt and pepper.
5. This savory breakfast is rich in healthy fats, protein, and a burst of freshness.

Recipe 3. Greek Yogurt Parfait with Nuts and Berries

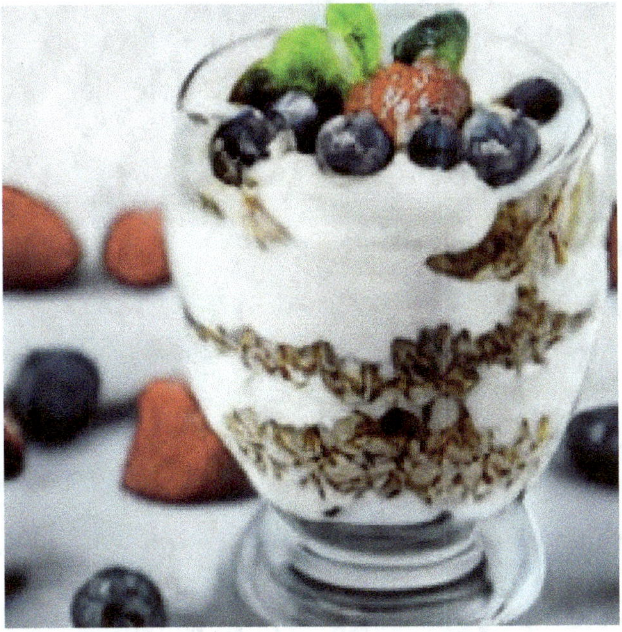

Ingredients:

- Greek yogurt
- Mixed berries (blueberries, strawberries, raspberries)
- Walnuts or almonds, chopped
- Honey
- Granola (optional)

Preparation:

1. Layer Greek yogurt with mixed berries in a glass.
2. Garnish with toasted, chopped nuts and a thread of honey.
3. Add granola for extra crunch if desired.
4. This parfait is a protein-packed, nutrient-rich delight to energize your morning.

Recipe 4. Spinach and Feta Omelette

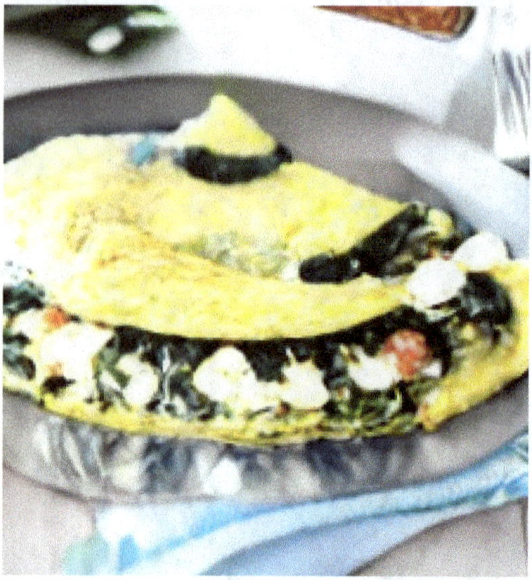

Ingredients:

- Eggs, beaten
- Fresh spinach, chopped
- Feta cheese, crumbled
- Cherry tomatoes, diced
- Olive oil
- Salt and pepper to taste

Preparation:

1. Sauté fresh spinach and diced cherry tomatoes in olive oil until wilted.
2. Pour beaten eggs over the vegetables.
3. Sprinkle crumbled feta cheese on one half of the omelet.
4. Gently bring the edges of the omelette together to form a half-moon shape and continue cooking until the eggs are fully set through.
5. Season with salt and pepper.
6. This savory omelette is a protein-packed breakfast option with a flavorful twist.

Recipe 5. Whole-grain pancakes with Mixed Berry Compote

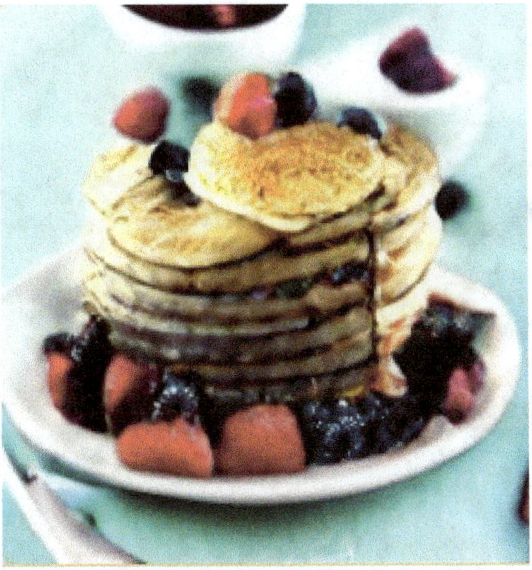

Ingredients:

- Whole-grain pancake mix
- Water or low-phosphorus milk
- Mixed berries (strawberries, blueberries, blackberries)
- Lemon juice
- Maple syrup

Preparation:

1. Prepare whole-grain pancakes according to the package instructions.
2. In a saucepan, simmer mixed berries with a splash of water, lemon juice, and a touch of maple syrup until it forms a compote.
3. Top the pancakes with the mixed berry compote.
4. Drizzle with additional maple syrup if desired.
5. These whole-grain pancakes offer a comforting and fiber-rich breakfast option..

Kidney-Friendly Pancakes and Waffles

Recipe 1. Whole-Grain Banana Pancakes

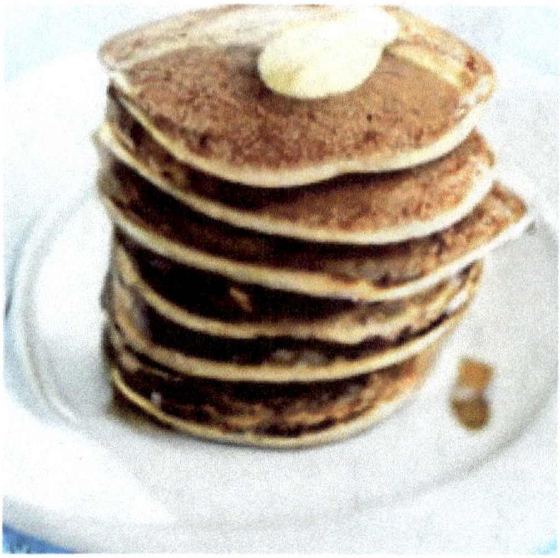

Ingredients:

- Whole-grain pancake mix
- Ripe bananas, mashed
- Low-phosphorus milk or water
- Cinnamon
- Vanilla extract
- Maple syrup (optional)

Preparation:

1. In a bowl, mix whole-grain pancake mix with mashed bananas, low-phosphorus milk or water, a dash of cinnamon, and a splash of vanilla extract.
2. Cook pancakes on a griddle or skillet.
3. Serve with a drizzle of maple syrup if desired.
4. These pancakes offer a wholesome, fiber-rich start to your morning.

Recipe 2. Sweet Potato Waffles

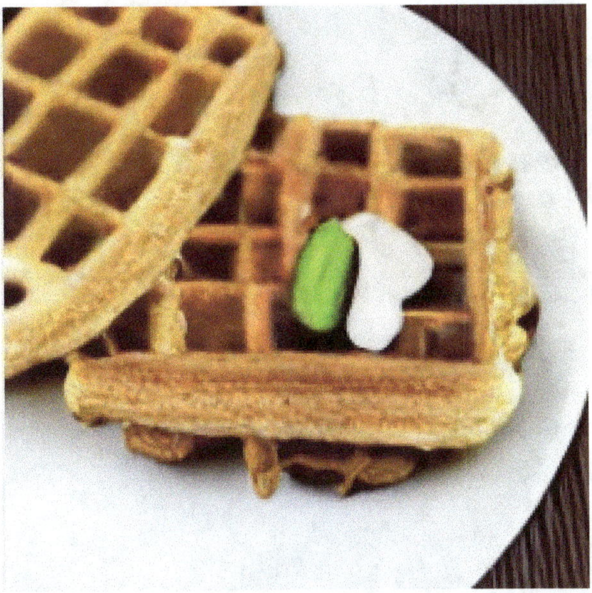

Ingredients:

- Sweet potatoes, cooked and mashed
- Whole-grain waffle mix
- Low-phosphorus milk or water
- Ground cinnamon
- Nutmeg
- Pecans, chopped (optional)

Preparation:

1. Combine mashed sweet potatoes with whole-grain waffle mix, low-phosphorus milk or water, ground cinnamon, and a pinch of nutmeg.
2. Cook the waffles according to the waffle maker's instructions.
3. Top with chopped pecans for added crunch if desired.
4. These waffles are a delightful blend of sweet potatoes, whole grains, and warm spices.

Recipe 3. Blueberry Buckwheat Pancakes

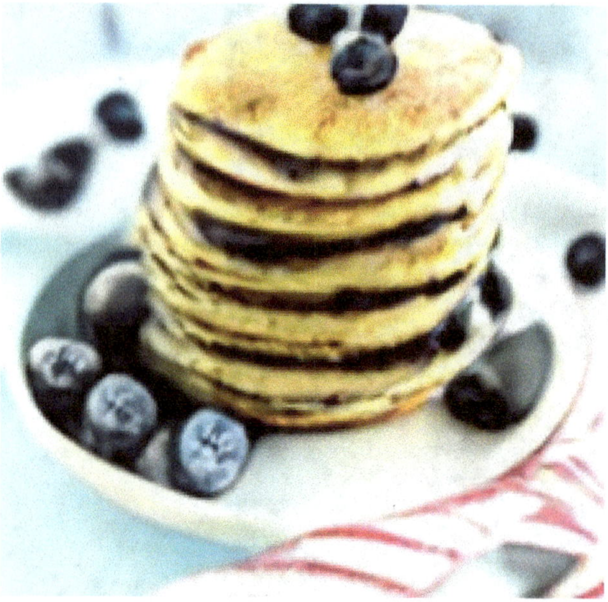

Ingredients:

- Buckwheat pancake mix
- Low-phosphorus milk or water
- Fresh blueberries
- Lemon zest
- Greek yogurt (optional)

Preparation:

1. Prepare buckwheat pancake mix with low-phosphorus milk or water.
2. Gently fold in fresh blueberries and a hint of lemon zest.
3. Cook pancakes on a griddle until golden brown.
4. Serve with a dollop of Greek yogurt for added creaminess if desired.
5. These blueberry buckwheat pancakes offer a burst of antioxidants and a satisfying texture.

Recipe 4. Cinnamon Apple Oat Waffles

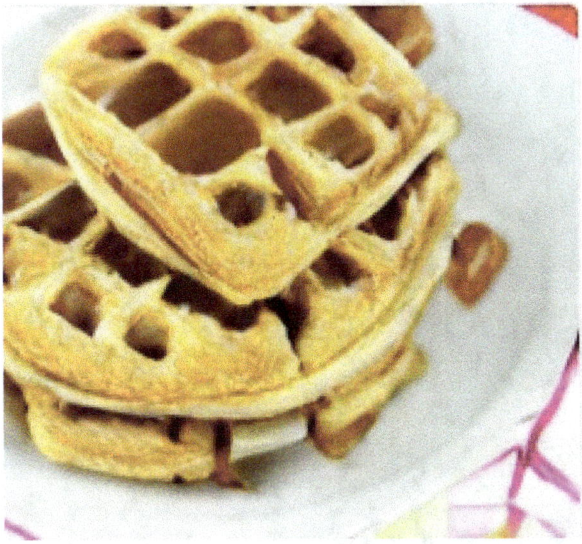

Ingredients:

- Oat waffle mix
- Low-phosphorus milk or water
- Apples, finely chopped
- Ground cinnamon
- Walnuts, chopped (optional)

Preparation:

1. Prepare oat waffle mix with low-phosphorus milk or water.
2. Fold in finely chopped apples and a generous sprinkle of ground cinnamon.
3. Cook the waffles in a waffle maker.
4. Top with chopped walnuts for an extra crunch if desired.
5. These cinnamon apple oat waffles are a delightful fusion of wholesome oats and sweet, crisp apples.

Recipe 5. Spinach and Feta Pancakes

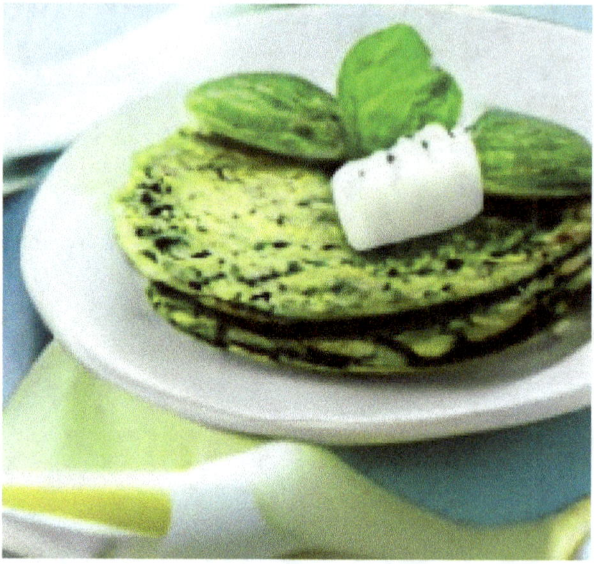

Ingredients:

- Whole-grain pancake mix
- Fresh spinach, chopped
- Feta cheese, crumbled
- Low-phosphorus milk or water
- Olive oil

Preparation:

1. Mix whole-grain pancake mix with chopped fresh spinach, crumbled feta cheese, and low-phosphorus milk or water.
2. Cook the pancakes on a griddle with a touch of olive oil.
3. Serve these savory pancakes with a side of Greek yogurt if desired.
4. These spinach and feta pancakes provide a savory twist to your morning routine.

Energizing Smoothies

Recipe 1. Berry Burst Green Smoothie

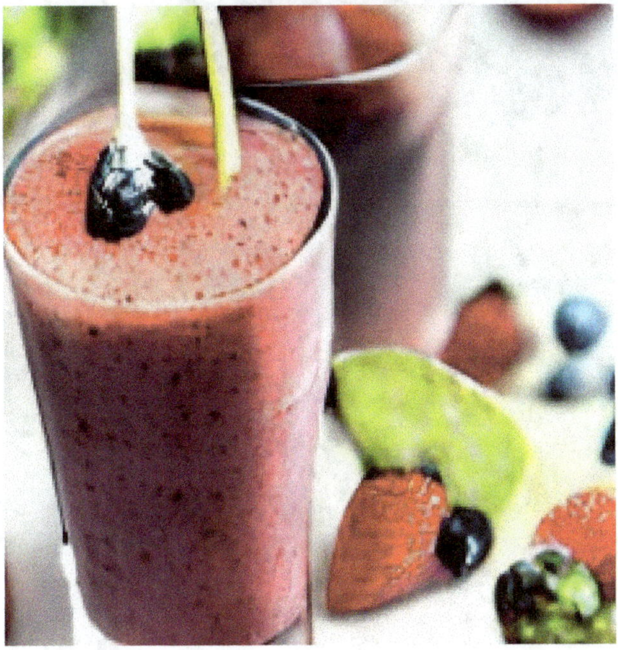

Ingredients:

- Spinach
- Mixed berries (strawberries, blueberries, raspberries)
- Banana
- Greek yogurt
- Almond milk
- Chia seeds
- Honey (optional)

Preparation:

1. Blend fresh spinach, mixed berries, banana, Greek yogurt, almond milk, and chia seeds until smooth.
2. Add honey for sweetness if desired.
3. This green smoothie is a powerhouse of antioxidants, vitamins, and plant-based protein.

Recipe 2. Tropical Citrus Splash

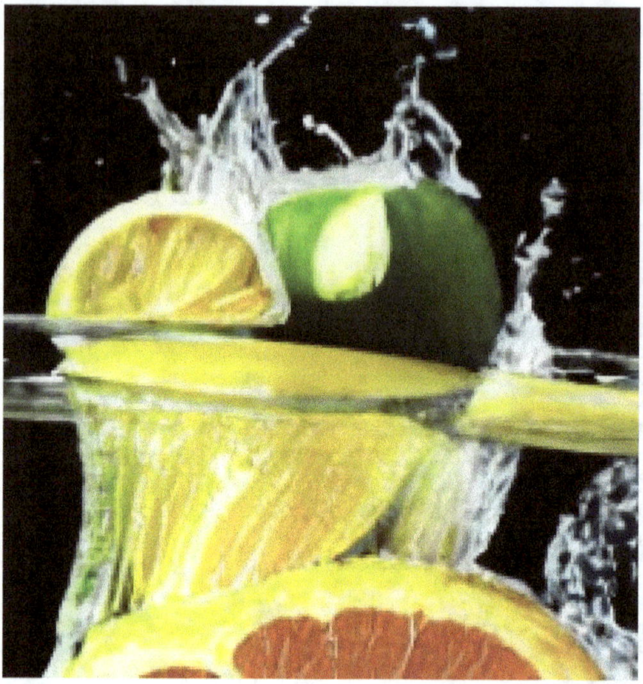

Ingredients:

- Pineapple chunks
- Mango slices
- Orange juice
- Greek yogurt
- Coconut water
- Ice cubes

Preparation:

1. Blend pineapple chunks, mango slices, orange juice, Greek yogurt, and coconut water until smooth.
2. Add ice cubes for a refreshing touch.
3. This tropical delight is rich in vitamin C, electrolytes, and a tropical burst of flavor.

Recipe 3. Coffee-Banana Protein Smoothie

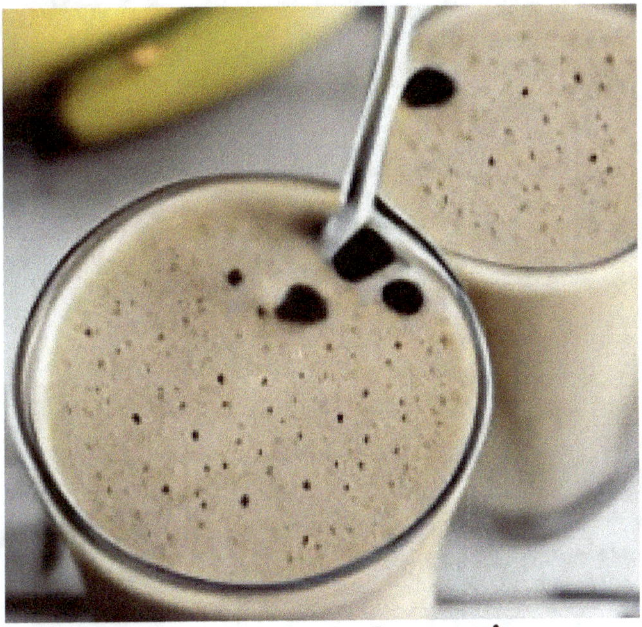

Ingredients:

- Cold brew coffee
- Banana
- Protein powder (low-phosphorus)
- Almond milk
- Ice cubes

Preparation:

1. Blend cold brew coffee, banana, low-phosphorus protein powder, almond milk, and ice cubes until smooth.
2. This smoothie offers a caffeinated kick, a protein boost, and a touch of sweetness.

Recipe 4. Green Tea-Berry Fusion

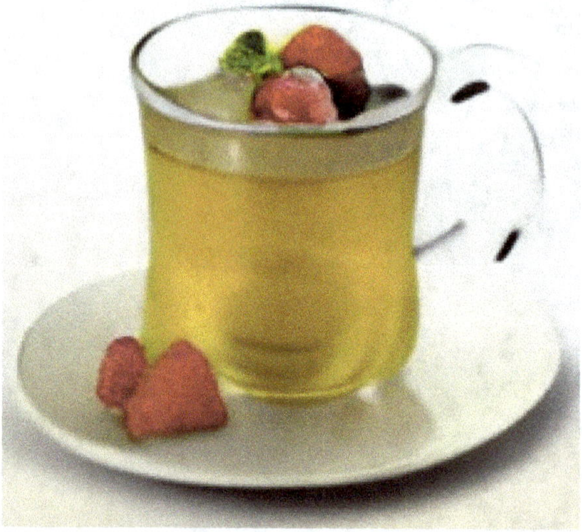

Ingredients:

- Green tea (cooled)
- Mixed berries (blueberries, strawberries, raspberries)
- Kale leaves
- Greek yogurt
- Honey
- Ice cubes

Preparation:

1. Blend cooled green tea, mixed berries, kale leaves, Greek yogurt, honey, and ice cubes until smooth.
2. The fusion of green tea and berries provides antioxidants and a refreshing zing..

Recipe 5. Creamy Avocado Spinach Smoothie

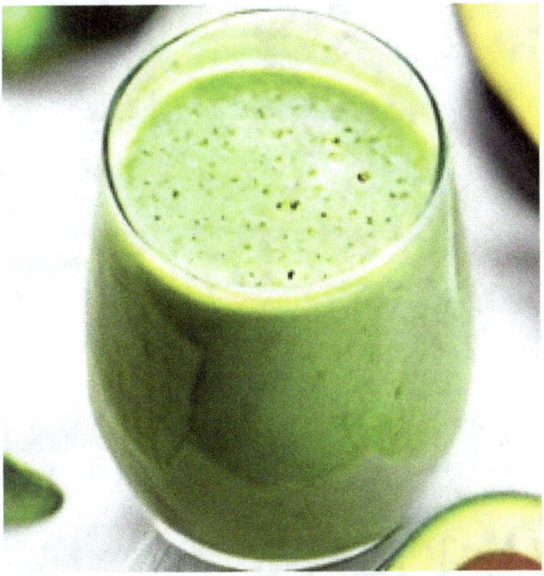

Ingredients:

- Avocado
- Fresh spinach leaves
- Banana
- Low-phosphorus milk or water
- Chia seeds
- Lime juice
- Ice cubes

Preparation:

1. Blend avocado, fresh spinach leaves, banana, low-phosphorus milk or water, chia seeds, lime juice, and ice cubes until creamy.
2. This smoothie offers a creamy texture, healthy fats, and a dose of vitamin C.

Recipe 6. Almond Butter and Banana Bliss

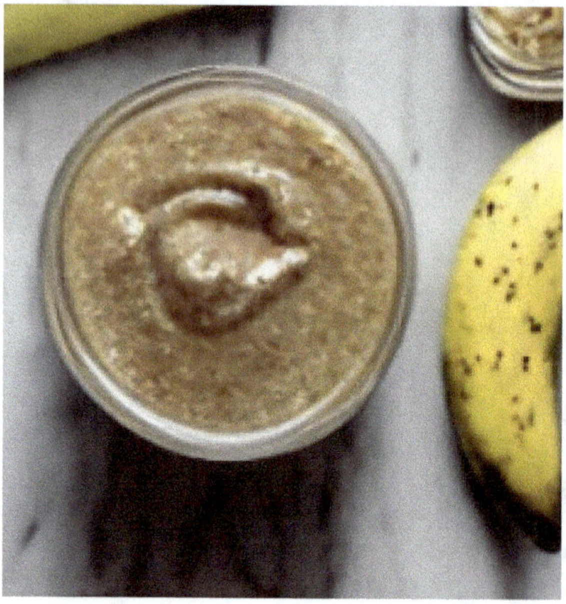

Ingredients:

- Banana
- Almond butter
- Low-phosphorus milk
- Greek yogurt
- Cinnamon
- Ice cubes

Preparation:

1. Blend banana, almond butter, low-phosphorus milk, Greek yogurt, cinnamon, and ice cubes until smooth.
2. This creamy delight provides a protein boost and a hint of nutty sweetness..

Chapter 5
Satisfying Lunches

Wholesome Salads and Soups

Recipe 1. Mediterranean Chickpea Salad

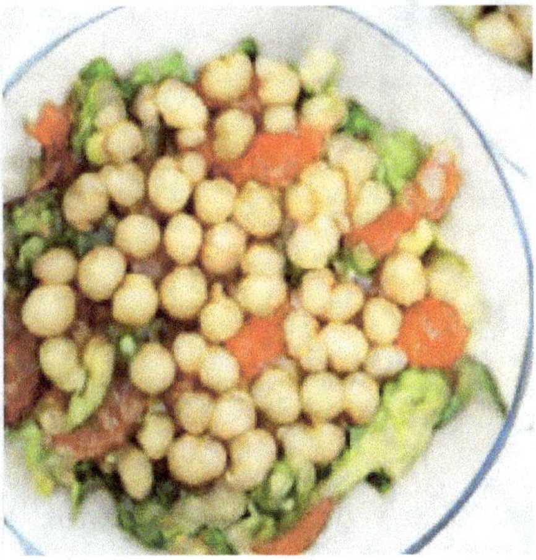

Ingredients:

- Chickpeas (canned, rinsed, and drained)
- Cucumber, diced
- Cherry tomatoes, halved
- Red onion, finely chopped
- Kalamata olives, sliced
- Feta cheese, crumbled
- Olive oil
- Lemon juice
- Fresh oregano, chopped
- Salt and pepper to taste

Preparation:

1. Combine chickpeas, cucumber, cherry tomatoes, red onion, olives, and feta cheese in a bowl.
2. Drizzle with olive oil and lemon juice.
3. Season with fresh oregano, salt, and pepper.
4. This Mediterranean delight is a satisfying blend of protein, fiber, and vibrant flavors.

Recipe 2. Quinoa and Vegetable Buddha Bowl

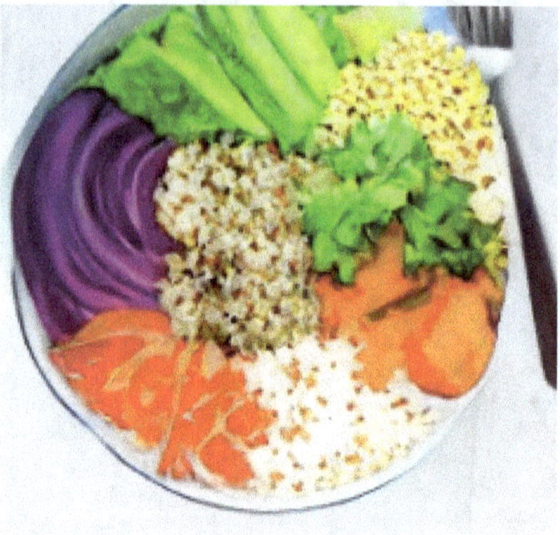

Ingredients:

- Quinoa, cooked
- Mixed vegetables (bell peppers, broccoli, carrots)
- Avocado, sliced
- Edamame steamed
- Sesame seeds
- Soy sauce
- Ginger, grated
- Green onions, chopped

Preparation:

1. Arrange cooked quinoa in a bowl.
2. Surround with a colorful array of mixed vegetables, sliced avocado, and steamed edamame.
3. Adorn the dish with toasted sesame seeds and a vibrant scattering of finely chopped green onions.
4. Drizzle with a mixture of soy sauce and grated ginger.
5. This Buddha Bowl is a wholesome combination of grains, vegetables, and plant-based protein.

Recipe 3. Chicken and Vegetable Stir-Fry with Brown Rice

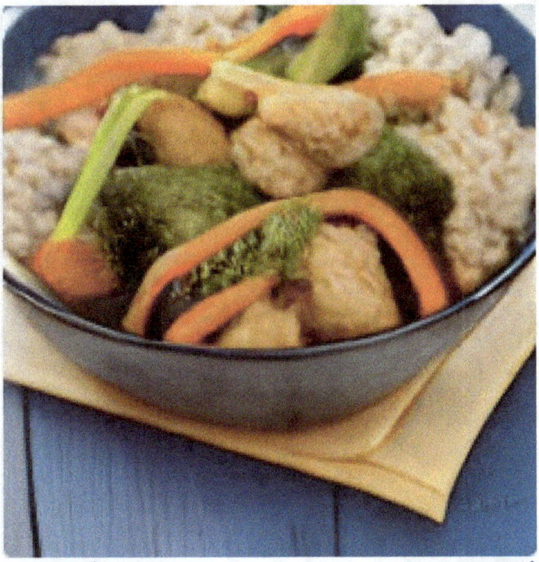

Ingredients:

- Boneless, skinless chicken breast, sliced
- Broccoli florets
- Bell peppers, sliced
- Carrots, julienned
- Low-sodium soy sauce
- Garlic, minced
- Ginger, grated
- Brown rice, cooked

Preparation:

1. Stir-fry sliced chicken until browned and fully cooked.
2. Add broccoli, bell peppers, carrots, minced garlic, and grated ginger to the pan.
3. Drizzle with low-sodium soy sauce and continue to stir-fry until vegetables are tender.
4. Serve over cooked brown rice.
5. This protein-packed stir-fry is a satisfying and savory lunch option.

Recipe 4. Tomato and Basil Quinoa Soup

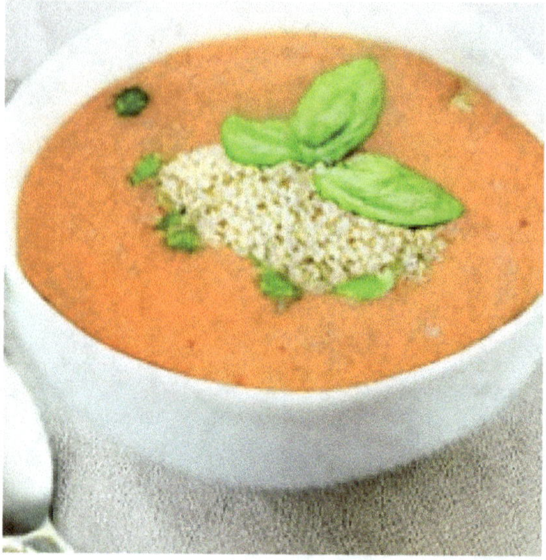

Ingredients:

- Quinoa, uncooked
- Tomatoes, diced
- Vegetable broth (low-sodium)
- Onion, diced
- Garlic, minced
- Fresh basil, chopped
- Olive oil
- Salt and pepper to taste

Preparation:

1. Sauté diced onion and minced garlic in olive oil until softened.
2. Add diced tomatoes, simmering until juices emerge.
3. Pour in low-sodium vegetable broth and bring to a simmer.
4. Add quinoa and cook until tender.
5. Stir in fresh basil, salt, and pepper.
6. This hearty quinoa soup is a comforting and nutrient-rich lunch option.

Recipe 5. Spinach and Lentil Salad

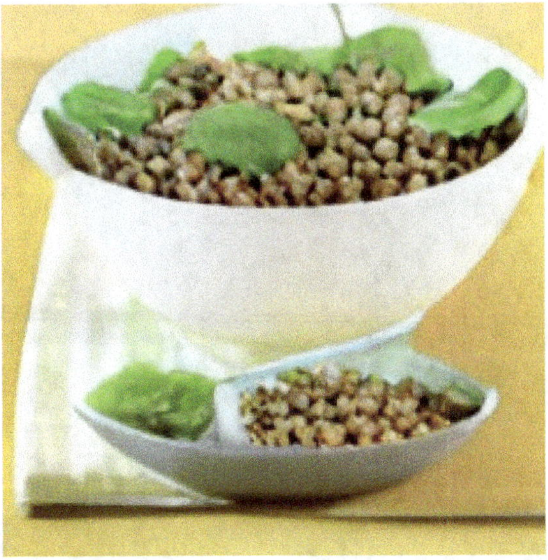

Ingredients:

- Lentils, cooked
- Fresh spinach leaves
- Cherry tomatoes, halved
- Red onion, thinly sliced
- Feta cheese, crumbled
- Balsamic vinaigrette dressing
- Walnuts, chopped (optional)

Preparation:

1. Toss together cooked lentils, fresh spinach, cherry tomatoes, sliced red onion, and crumbled feta cheese.
2. Drizzle with balsamic vinaigrette dressing.
3. Top with chopped walnuts if desired.
4. This salad is a delightful fusion of protein, iron, and a variety of textures.

Protein-Packed Sandwiches and Wraps

Recipe 1. Turkey and Avocado Wrap

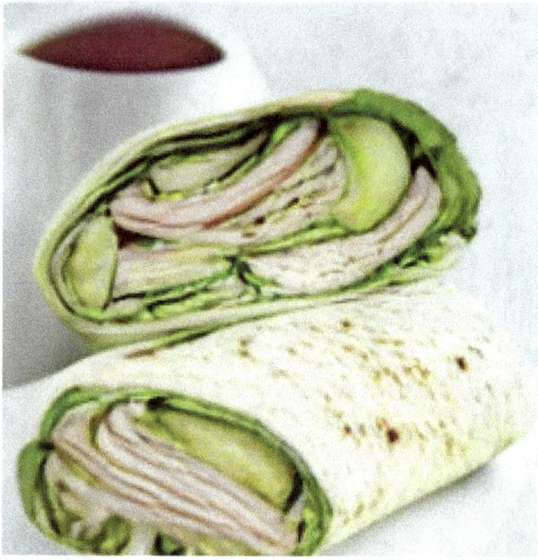

Ingredients:

- Whole-grain wrap
- Sliced turkey breast
- Avocado, sliced
- Tomato, sliced
- Leafy greens (lettuce or spinach)
- Greek yogurt spread
- Salt and pepper to taste

Preparation:

1. Lay out the whole-grain wrap and spread a layer of Greek yogurt.
2. Arrange sliced turkey, avocado, tomato, and leafy greens.
3. Season with salt and pepper to taste.
4. Roll the wrap tightly and slice it in half for a protein-packed delight.

Recipe 2. Grilled Chicken Caesar Wrap

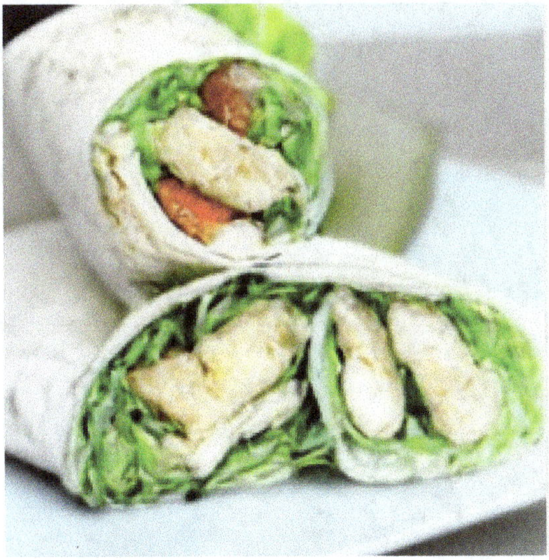

Ingredients:

- Whole-grain wrap
- Grilled chicken breast, sliced
- Romaine lettuce, chopped
- Cherry tomatoes, halved
- Parmesan cheese, shredded
- Caesar dressing (low-sodium)
- Black pepper to taste

Preparation:

1. Place grilled chicken slices on the whole-grain wrap.
2. Add chopped romaine lettuce, halved cherry tomatoes, and shredded Parmesan cheese.
3. Drizzle with low-sodium Caesar dressing.
4. Sprinkle black pepper to taste.
5. Roll the wrap and secure with a toothpick for a protein-packed Caesar sensation.

Recipe 3. Tuna Salad Lettuce Wraps

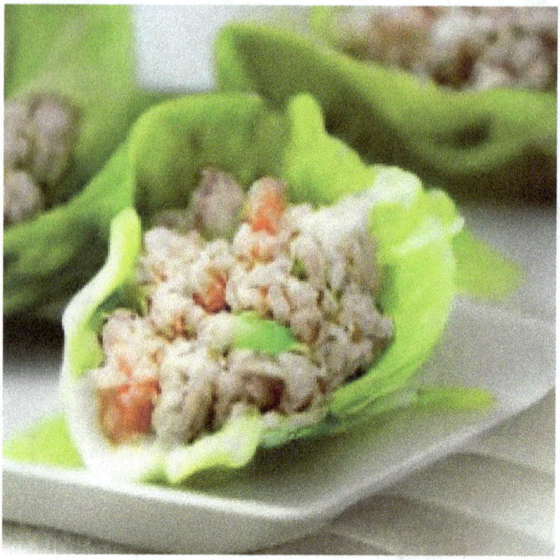

Ingredients:

- Canned tuna, drained
- Greek yogurt
- Celery, finely chopped
- Red onion, finely diced
- Dill, chopped
- Lettuce leaves (such as iceberg or butter lettuce)
- Lemon juice
- Salt and pepper to taste

Preparation:

1. In a bowl, mix canned tuna, Greek yogurt, chopped celery, diced red onion, and fresh dill.
2. Drizzle with lemon juice and season with salt and pepper.
3. Spoon the tuna salad onto lettuce leaves to create refreshing and protein-packed wraps.

Recipe 4. Egg Salad Sandwich

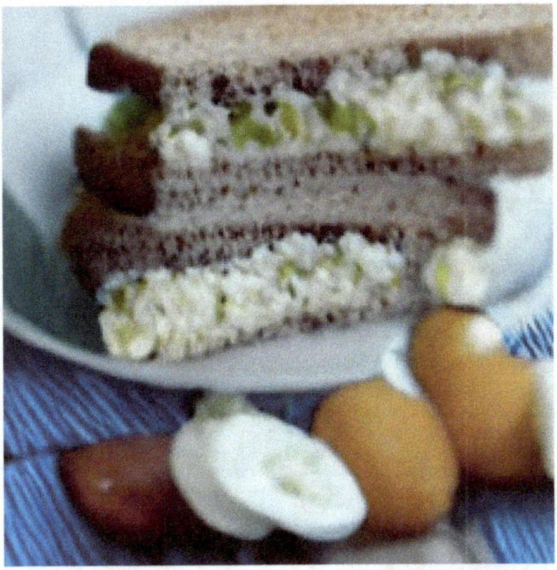

Ingredients:

- Hard-boiled eggs, chopped
- Greek yogurt
- Dijon mustard
- Celery, finely chopped
- Whole-grain bread
- Leafy greens (arugula or watercress)
- Salt and pepper to taste

Preparation:

1. Combine chopped hard-boiled eggs, Greek yogurt, Dijon mustard, and chopped celery in a bowl.
2. Spread the mixture on whole-grain bread.
3. Top with leafy greens and season with salt and pepper.
4. This egg salad sandwich offers a protein-rich twist on a classic favorite.

Recipe 5. Hummus and Veggie Wrap

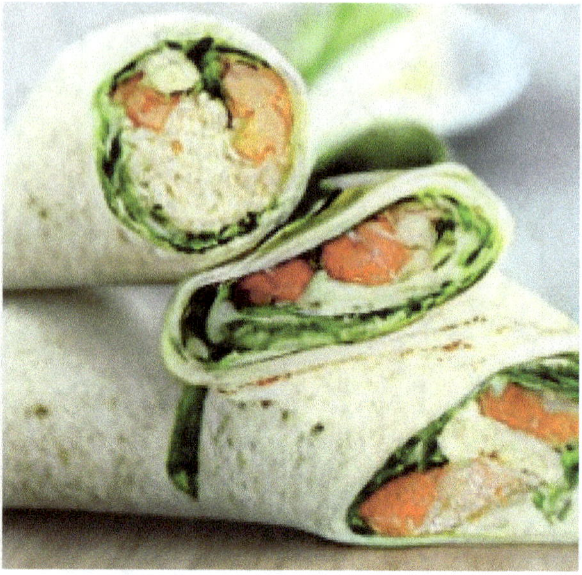

Ingredients:

- Whole-grain wrap
- Hummus
- Cherry tomatoes, sliced
- Cucumber, thinly sliced
- Red bell pepper, thinly sliced
- Red onion, thinly sliced
- Fresh parsley, chopped
- Olive oil
- Salt and pepper to taste

Preparation:

1. Spread a generous layer of hummus on the whole-grain wrap.
2. Arrange sliced cherry tomatoes, cucumber, red bell pepper, and red onion.
3. Sprinkle with chopped fresh parsley.
4. Drizzle with olive oil and season with salt and pepper.
5. Roll the wrap for a satisfying and protein-packed veggie delight.

Recipe 6. Black Bean and Avocado Quesadilla

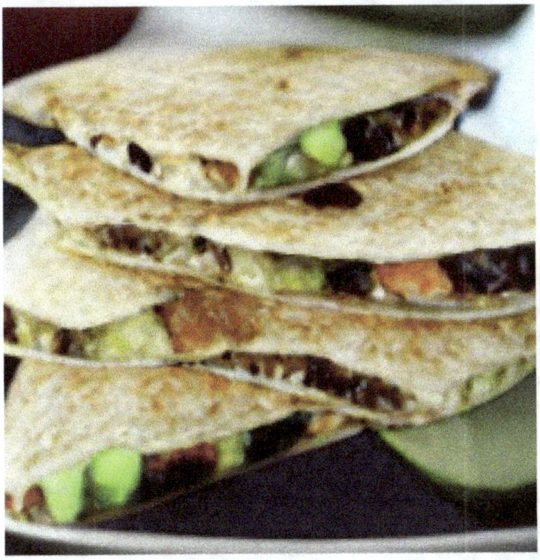

Ingredients:

- Whole-grain tortillas
- Black beans, cooked and mashed
- Avocado, mashed
- Shredded low-phosphorus cheese
- Salsa (low-sodium)
- Fresh cilantro, chopped

Preparation:

1. Spread mashed black beans and avocado on a whole-grain tortilla.
2. Sprinkle with shredded low-phosphorus cheese and top with salsa.
3. Place another tortilla on top and press down gently.
4. Cook in a skillet until the tortilla is crispy and the cheese is melted.
5. Garnish with chopped fresh cilantro and slice into wedges for a protein-packed quesadilla.

Flavorful Grain Bowls

Recipe 1. Quinoa and Roasted Vegetable Bowl

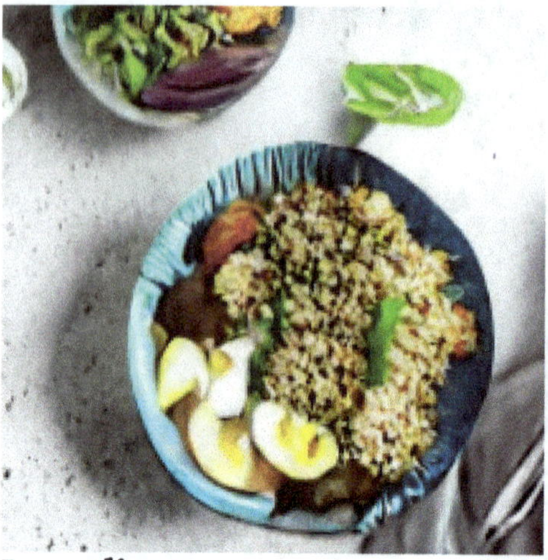

Ingredients:

- Quinoa, cooked
- Sweet potatoes, diced
- Bell peppers, sliced
- Red onion, wedges
- Cherry tomatoes, halved
- Olive oil
- Garlic powder
- Paprika
- Fresh cilantro, chopped
- Lemon wedges

Preparation:

1. Roast sweet potatoes, bell peppers, red onion, and cherry tomatoes in olive oil, garlic powder, and paprika until tender.
2. Arrange the roasted vegetables over a bed of cooked quinoa.
3. Sprinkle with fresh cilantro and serve with lemon wedges for a zesty touch.
4. This grain bowl is a colorful medley of flavors and textures.

Recipe 2. Brown Rice and Teriyaki Tofu Bowl

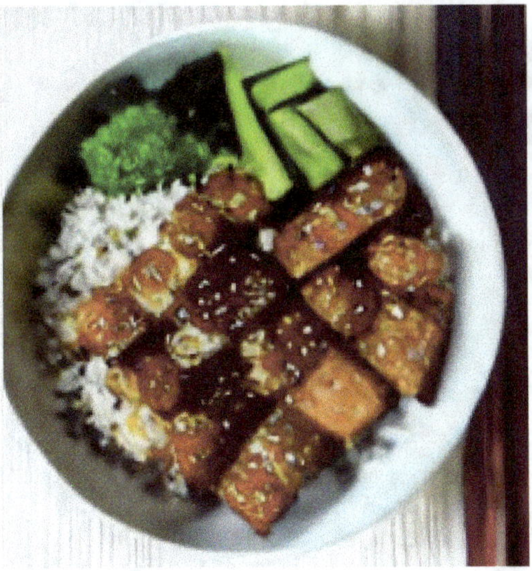

Ingredients:

- Brown rice, cooked
- Extra-firm tofu, cubed and sautéed in teriyaki sauce
- Broccoli florets, steamed
- Carrots, julienned
- Edamame steamed
- Sesame seeds
- Green onions, sliced

Preparation:

1. Layer cooked brown rice with teriyaki tofu, steamed broccoli, julienned carrots, and edamame.
2. Garnish with toasted sesame seeds and thinly sliced green onions.
3. Drizzle with additional teriyaki sauce if desired.
4. This bowl is a savory fusion of protein-packed tofu and wholesome grains.

Recipe 3. Mediterranean Farro Bowl

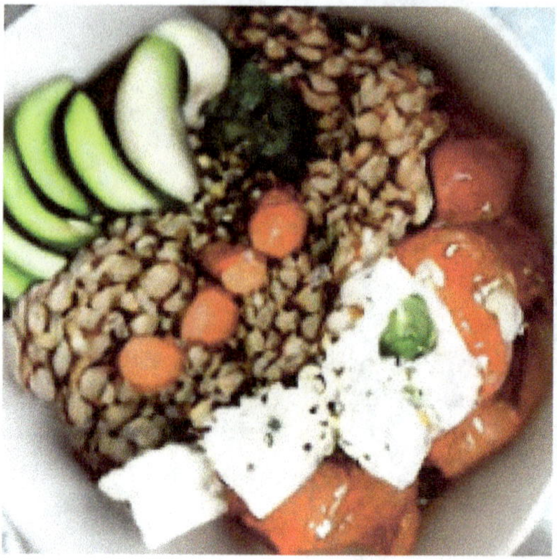

Ingredients:

- Farro, cooked
- Grilled chicken breast, sliced
- Cucumber, diced
- Kalamata olives, sliced
- Cherry tomatoes, halved
- Feta cheese, crumbled
- Fresh dill, chopped
- Greek dressing

Preparation:

1. Combine cooked farro with grilled chicken, diced cucumber, sliced olives, halved cherry tomatoes, and crumbled feta cheese.
2. Toss with fresh dill and drizzle with Greek dressing.
3. This Mediterranean-inspired bowl is a symphony of flavors and a source of lean protein.

Recipe 4. Wild Rice and Salmon Bowl

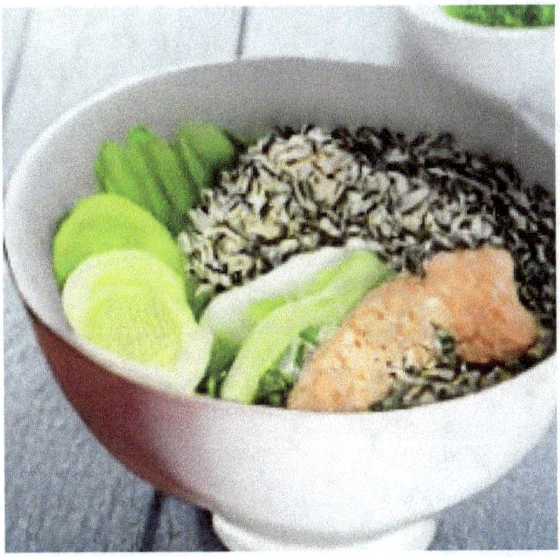

Ingredients:

- Wild rice, cooked
- Baked salmon fillet, flaked
- Asparagus spears, roasted
- Avocado, sliced
- Radishes, thinly sliced
- Lemon-dill vinaigrette
- Fresh parsley, chopped

Preparation:

1. Arrange cooked wild rice with flaked salmon, roasted asparagus, sliced avocado, and thinly sliced radishes.
2. Drizzle with lemon-dill vinaigrette.
3. Adorn the dish with a chiffonade of fresh parsley for an enlivening accent.
4. This bowl is a delightful combination of omega-3-rich salmon and hearty wild rice.

Recipe 5. Black Bean and Brown Rice Fiesta Bowl

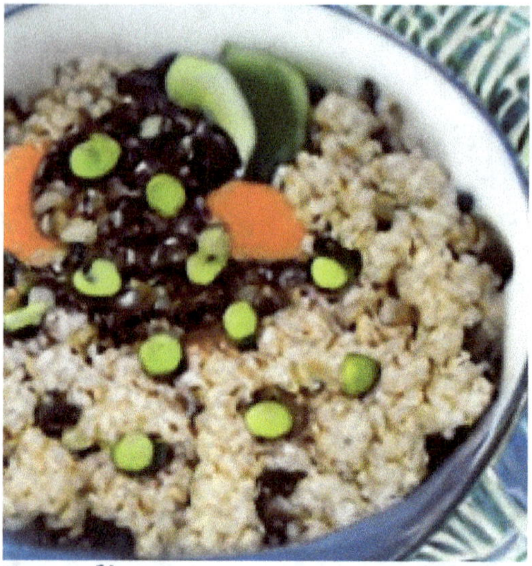

Ingredients:

- Wild rice, cooked
- Baked salmon fillet, flaked
- Asparagus spears, roasted
- Avocado, sliced
- Radishes, thinly sliced
- Lemon-dill vinaigrette
- Fresh parsley, chopped

Preparation:

1. Arrange cooked wild rice with flaked salmon, roasted asparagus, sliced avocado, and thinly sliced radishes.
2. Drizzle with lemon-dill vinaigrette.
3. Adorn the dish with a chiffonade of fresh parsley for an enlivening accent.
4. This bowl is a delightful combination of omega-3-rich salmon and hearty wild rice.

Recipe 5. Black Bean and Brown Rice Fiesta Bowl

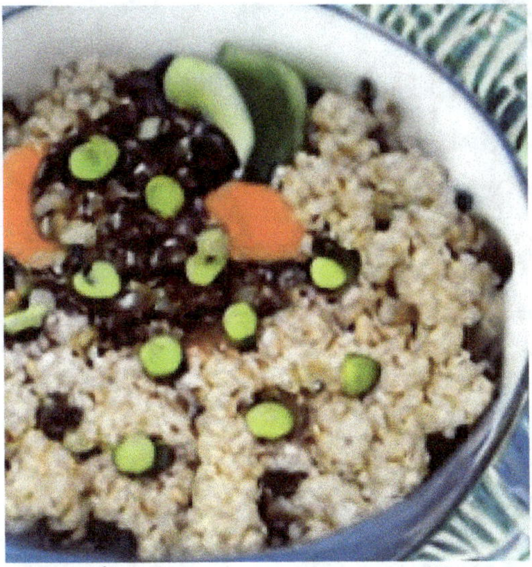

Ingredients:

- Brown rice, cooked
- Black beans, cooked
- Corn kernels, grilled
- Red bell pepper, diced
- Jalapeño, sliced
- Avocado, diced
- Lime wedges
- Cilantro-lime dressing

Preparation:

1. Combine cooked brown rice with black beans, grilled corn, diced red bell pepper, and sliced jalapeño.
2. Add diced avocado and serve with lime wedges.
3. Drizzle with cilantro-lime dressing for a zesty kick.
4. This fiesta bowl is a celebration of colors and Southwestern flavors.

Recipe 6. Spinach and Chickpea Quinoa Bowl

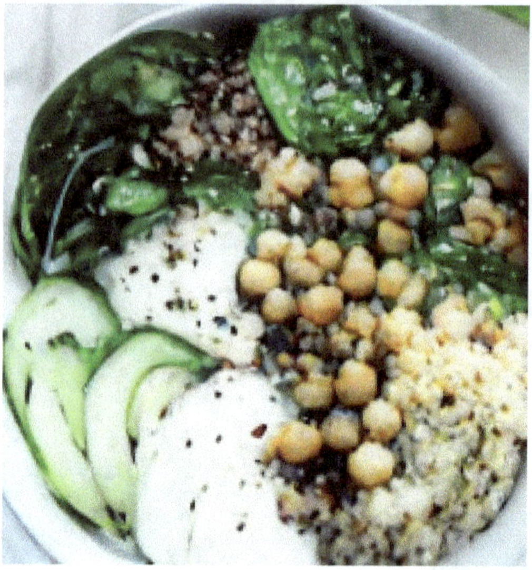

Ingredients:

- Quinoa, cooked
- Chickpeas, roasted
- Fresh spinach leaves
- Red onion, thinly sliced
- Cherry tomatoes, halved
- Cucumber, diced
- Tahini dressing

Preparation:

1. Layer cooked quinoa with roasted chickpeas, fresh spinach leaves, thinly sliced red onion, halved cherry tomatoes, and diced cucumber.
2. Drizzle with tahini dressing for a creamy finish.
3. This bowl is a wholesome blend of protein-rich chickpeas and nutrient-packed vegetables.

Chapter 6
Nourishing Dinners

Delicious One-Pot Meals

Recipe 1. Lemon Herb Chicken and Vegetable Skillet

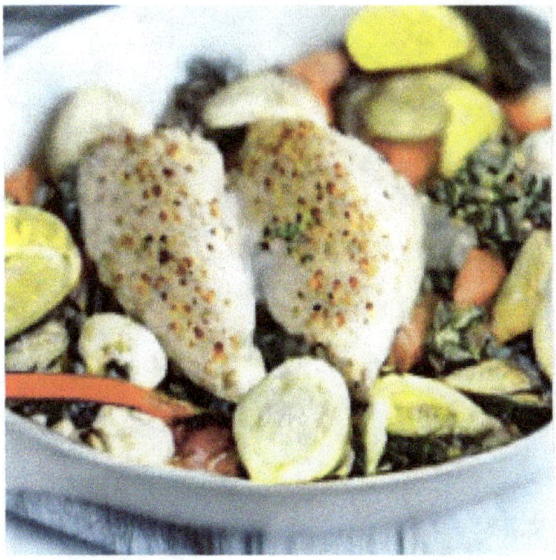

Ingredients:

- Boneless, skinless chicken thighs
- Baby potatoes, halved
- Carrots, sliced
- Green beans, trimmed
- Garlic, minced
- Lemon zest
- Fresh thyme
- Olive oil
- Salt and pepper to taste

Preparation:

1. Sear chicken thighs in olive oil until browned.
2. Add halved baby potatoes, sliced carrots, trimmed green beans, minced garlic, lemon zest, and fresh thyme to the skillet.
3. Season with salt and pepper.
4. Cover and let simmer until the chicken is cooked through and vegetables are tender.
5. This one-pot wonder is a zesty and herb-infused delight.

Recipe 2. Shrimp and Broccoli Stir-Fry Rice

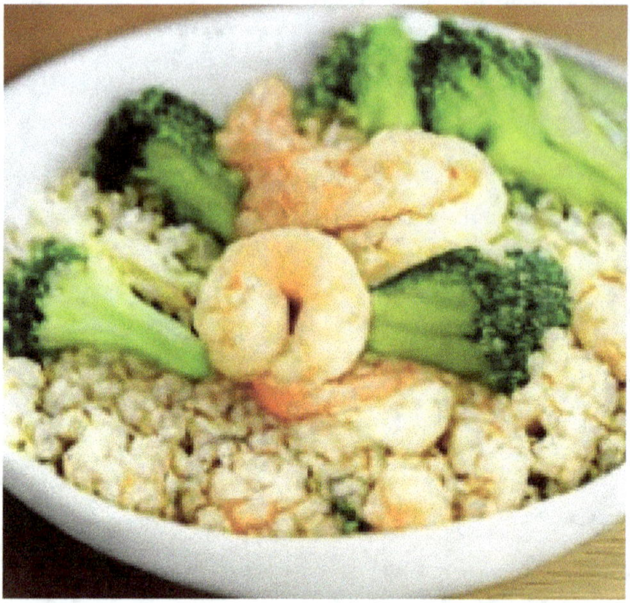

Ingredients:

- Brown rice, cooked
- Shrimp, peeled and deveined
- Broccoli florets
- Bell peppers, sliced
- Soy sauce (low-sodium)
- Ginger, grated
- Garlic, minced
- Sesame oil
- Green onions, sliced

Preparation:

1. Sauté shrimp in sesame oil until cooked.
2. Add broccoli florets, sliced bell peppers, grated ginger, and minced garlic to the skillet.
3. Stir in cooked brown rice and soy sauce.
4. Cook until vegetables are tender.
5. Garnish with sliced green onions for a quick and flavorful stir-fry.

Recipe 3. Beef and Vegetable Quinoa Skillet

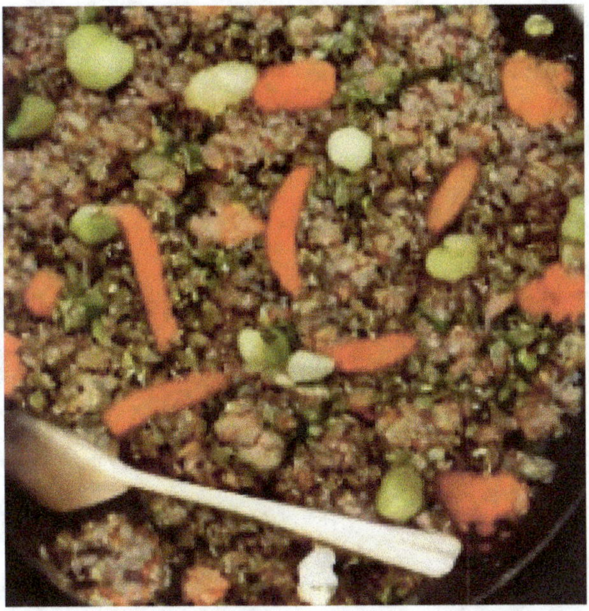

Ingredients:

- Lean ground beef
- Quinoa, uncooked
- Zucchini, diced
- Bell peppers, diced
- Onion, diced
- Crushed tomatoes
- Italian seasoning
- Parmesan cheese, grated
- Fresh basil, chopped

Preparation:

1. Brown lean ground beef in a skillet.
2. Add diced zucchini, bell peppers, and onion to the skillet.
3. Stir in uncooked quinoa, crushed tomatoes, and Italian seasoning.
4. Bring to a simmer and hold until quinoa has absorbed the liquid and vegetables are tender.
5. Top with grated Parmesan cheese and fresh basil for an Italian-inspired one-pot meal.

Recipe 4. Lentil and Vegetable Stew

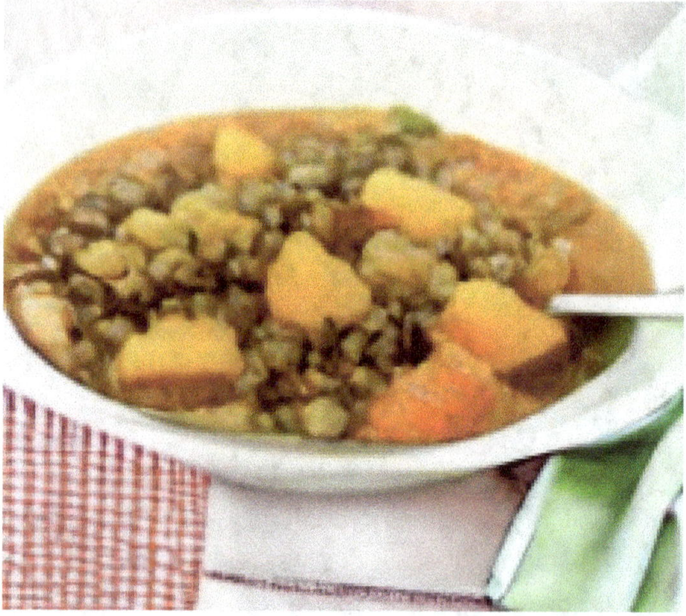

Ingredients:

- Green or brown lentils, uncooked
- Carrots, diced
- Celery, chopped
- Onion, finely chopped
- Garlic, minced
- Vegetable broth (low-sodium)
- Crushed tomatoes
- Cumin, ground
- Paprika
- Fresh parsley, chopped

Preparation:

1. Heat the diced onion and minced garlic in a skillet until they become tender.
2. Add uncooked lentils, diced carrots, chopped celery, crushed tomatoes, vegetable broth, ground cumin, and paprika to the pot.
3. Simmer until lentils are tender and vegetables are cooked.
4. Garnish with fresh parsley for a hearty and nutritious lentil stew.

Recipe 5. Salmon and Asparagus Foil Packets

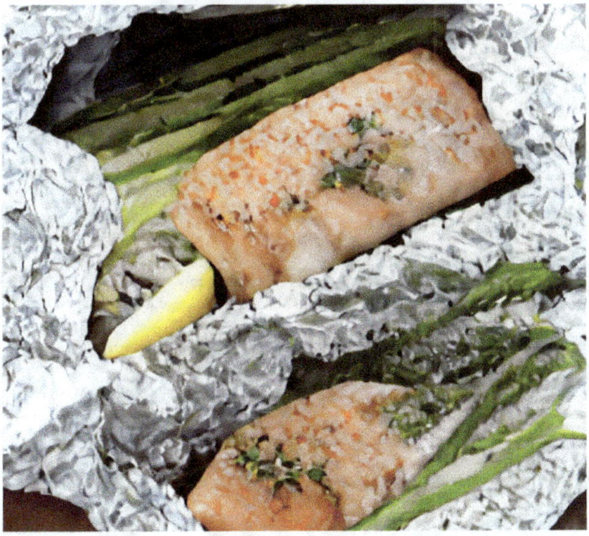

Ingredients:

- Salmon fillets
- Asparagus spears
- Cherry tomatoes, halved
- Lemon slices
- Garlic, minced
- Olive oil
- Dill, chopped
- Salt and pepper to taste

Preparation:

1. Place salmon fillets on a sheet of foil.
2. Add asparagus spears and halved cherry tomatoes around the salmon.
3. Drizzle with olive oil and sprinkle minced garlic, chopped dill, salt, and pepper.
4. Wrap the salmon tightly in foil, forming sealed packets. and bake until the salmon is cooked through.
5. These foil packets are a hassle-free way to enjoy a flavorful and nutritious dinner.

Recipe 6. Chickpea and Spinach Curry

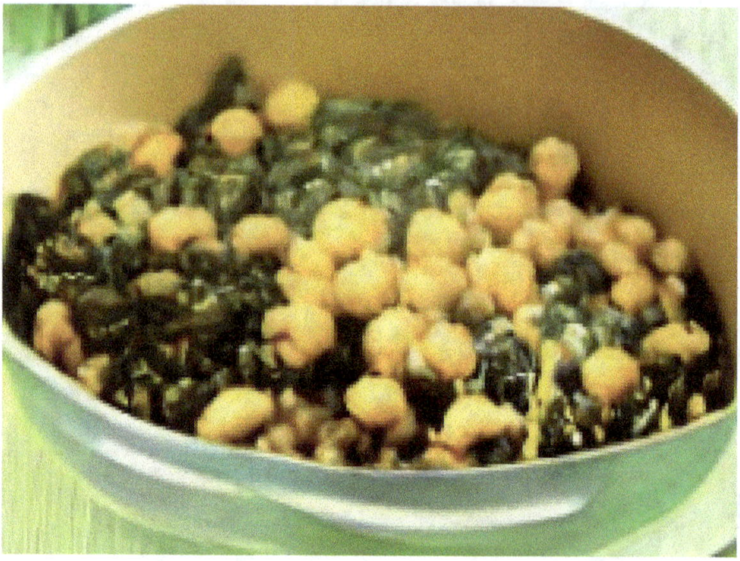

Ingredients:

- Chickpeas, cooked
- Fresh spinach leaves
- Onion, finely chopped
- Garlic, minced
- Ginger, grated
- Coconut milk
- Curry powder
- Turmeric
- Cilantro, chopped
- Basmati rice, cooked

Preparation:

1. Place salmon fillets on a sheet Sauté finely chopped onion, minced garlic, and grated ginger until fragrant.
2. Add cooked chickpeas, fresh spinach leaves, coconut milk, curry powder, and turmeric.
3. Simmer until the spinach wilts and the flavors meld.
4. Serve over cooked basmati rice and garnish with chopped cilantro for a satisfying chickpea curry.

Oven-Baked Goodness

Recipe 1. Herb-Crusted Baked Chicken Breast

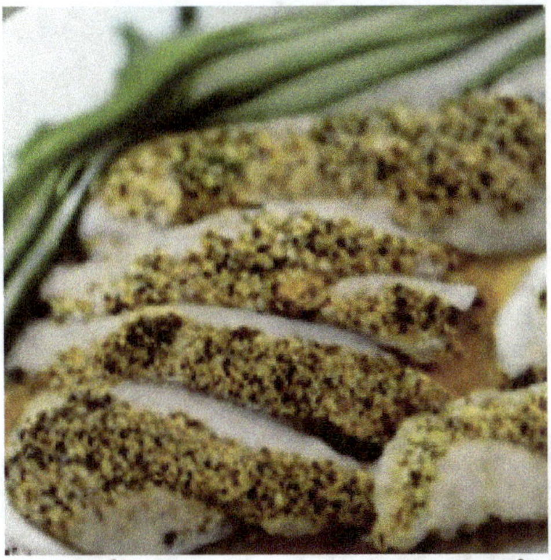

Ingredients:

- Boneless, skinless chicken breasts
- Fresh herbs (rosemary, thyme, parsley), chopped
- Garlic, minced
- Olive oil
- Lemon juice
- Salt and pepper to taste

Preparation:

1. Preheat the oven to the desired temperature before you begin.
2. In a bowl, mix chopped fresh herbs, minced garlic, olive oil, lemon juice, salt, and pepper.
3. Coat chicken breasts with the herb mixture and place them in the baking dish.
4. Bake until the internal temperature of the thickest part of the chicken reaches 165°F (74°C) and the skin achieves a deep golden brown.
5. This herb-crusted chicken is a fragrant and flavorful centerpiece for a wholesome meal.

Recipe 2. Baked Salmon with Lemon and Dill

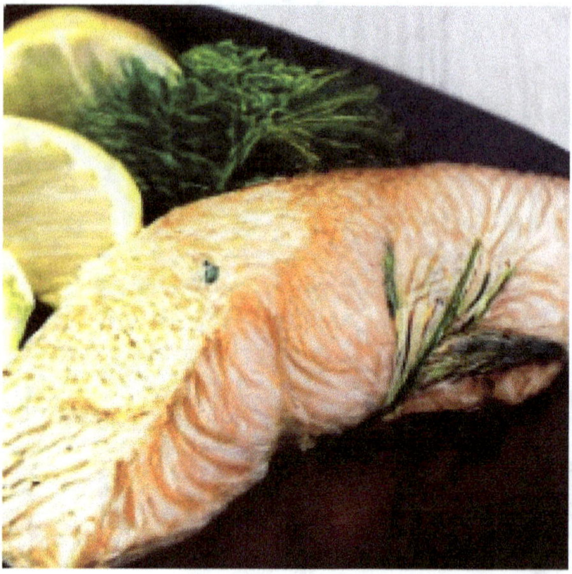

Ingredients:

- Salmon fillets
- Lemon slices
- Fresh dill, chopped
- Olive oil
- Garlic powder
- Salt and pepper to taste

Preparation:

1. Preheat the oven and place the salmon fillets on a baking sheet.
2. Arrange lemon slices on top of the salmon.
3. Drizzle with olive oil, sprinkle chopped fresh dill, garlic powder, salt, and pepper.
4. Bake until the salmon flakes easily when gently prodded with a fork.
5. This baked salmon is a refreshing and nutritious choice for seafood enthusiasts.

Recipe 3. Roasted Vegetable Medley

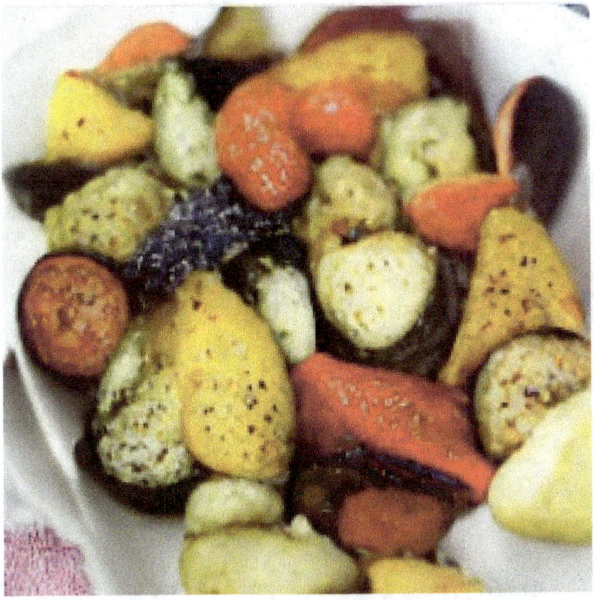

Ingredients:

- Assorted vegetables (bell peppers, zucchini, cherry tomatoes, carrots), chopped
- Olive oil
- Balsamic vinegar
- Garlic, minced
- Italian seasoning
- Salt and pepper to taste

Preparation:

1. Preheat the oven and spread chopped vegetables on a baking sheet.
2. Drizzle with olive oil and balsamic vinegar.
3. Sprinkle minced garlic, Italian seasoning, salt, and pepper.
4. Roast until the vegetables are caramelized and tender.
5. An artful symphony of roasted vegetables, this side dish delights both eye and palate.

Recipe 4. Sweet Potato and Chickpea Bake

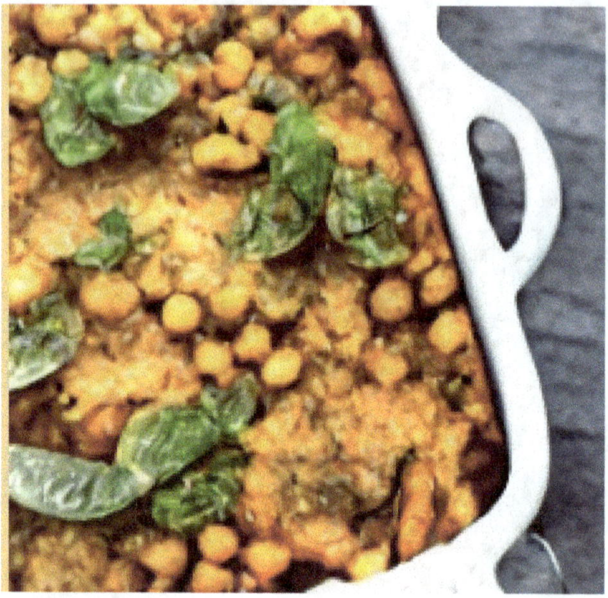

Ingredients:

- Sweet potatoes, peeled and diced
- Canned chickpeas, drained and rinsed
- Olive oil
- Cumin
- Paprika
- Garlic powder
- Salt and pepper to taste

Preparation:

1. Preheat the oven and toss diced sweet potatoes and chickpeas with olive oil.
2. Sprinkle with cumin, paprika, garlic powder, salt, and pepper.
3. Roast until sweet potatoes are golden and chickpeas are crispy.
4. This sweet potato and chickpea bake is a nutritious and satisfying dish.

Recipe 5. Baked Eggplant Parmesan

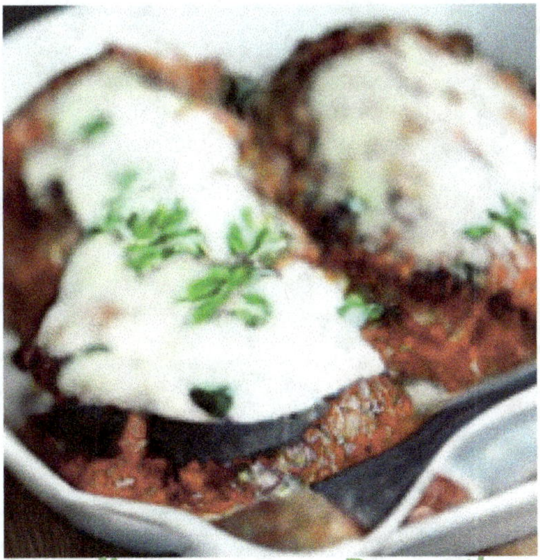

Ingredients:

- Eggplant, sliced
- Egg whites
- Whole-wheat breadcrumbs
- Marinara sauce (low-sodium)
- Mozzarella cheese, shredded
- Parmesan cheese, grated
- Fresh basil, chopped

Preparation:

1. Preheat the oven and dip eggplant slices in egg whites, then coat with whole-wheat breadcrumbs.
2. Place breaded eggplant on a baking sheet and bake until golden.
3. Layer baked eggplant with marinara sauce, mozzarella cheese, and Parmesan cheese.
4. Heat until the cheese achieves a state of complete melting and exhibits visible signs of bubbling activity.
5. Garnish with chopped fresh basil for a delightful baked eggplant Parmesan.

Recipe 6. Baked Stuffed Bell Peppers

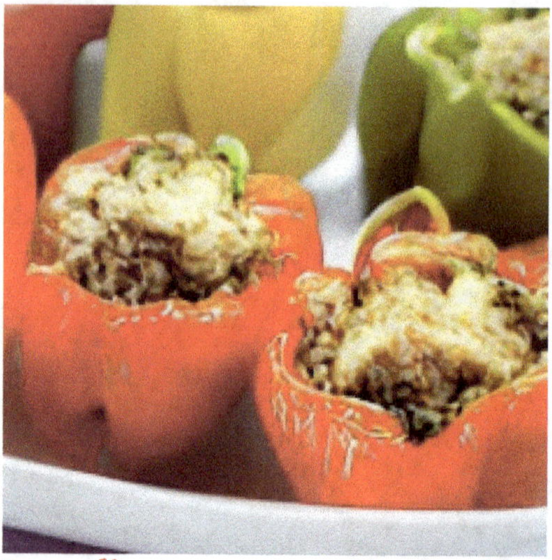

Ingredients:

- Bell peppers, halved
- Lean ground turkey
- Quinoa, cooked
- Black beans, drained and rinsed
- Corn kernels
- Salsa (low-sodium)
- Cumin
- Chili powder
- Shredded cheddar cheese

Preparation:

1. Heat oven. Place halved peppers in dish.
2. In a bowl, mix cooked quinoa, lean ground turkey, black beans, corn, salsa, cumin, and chili powder.
3. Fill each bell pepper half with the flavorful mix.
4. Top with shredded cheddar cheese and bake until peppers are tender.
5. These baked stuffed bell peppers are a flavorful and protein-packed meal.

Recipe 7. Apple Cinnamon Baked Oatmeal

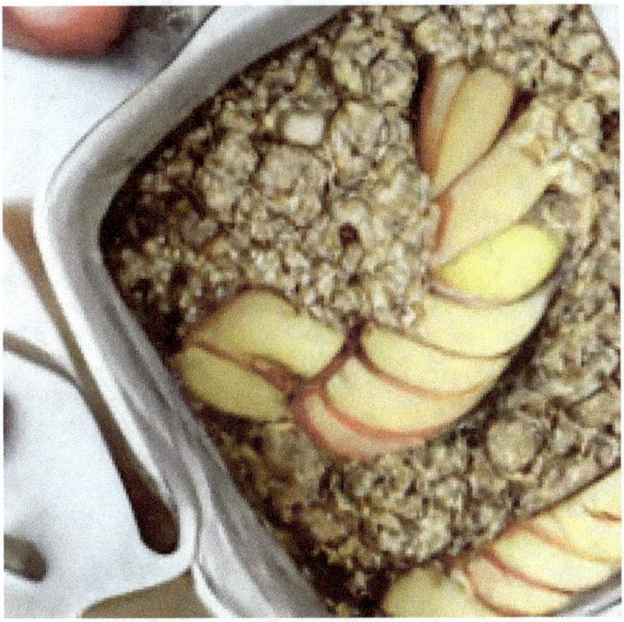

Ingredients:

- Rolled oats
- Apple diced
- Cinnamon
- Almond milk
- Maple syrup
- Walnuts, chopped
- Vanilla extract

Preparation:

1. Preheat the oven and mix rolled oats, diced apple, cinnamon, almond milk, maple syrup, chopped walnuts, and vanilla extract in a baking dish.
2. Bake until the oats are cooked and the top is golden.
3. This apple cinnamon baked oatmeal is a comforting and nutritious breakfast or dessert option.

Grilled Delights for Kidney Health

Recipe 1. Lemon Herb Grilled Chicken Breast

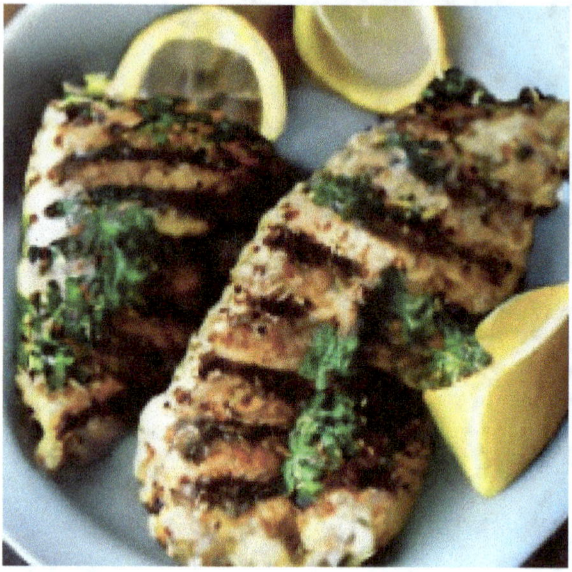

Ingredients:

- Chicken breasts, boneless and skinless
- Lemon juice
- Olive oil
- Fresh rosemary, chopped
- Garlic, minced
- Salt and pepper to taste

Preparation:

1. Marinate chicken breasts in a mixture of lemon juice, olive oil, chopped rosemary, minced garlic, salt, and pepper.
2. Grill until the chicken is cooked through and has a beautiful char.
3. This lemon herb grilled chicken is a lean and protein-packed option for a kidney-friendly meal.

Recipe 2. Balsamic Glazed Grilled Salmon

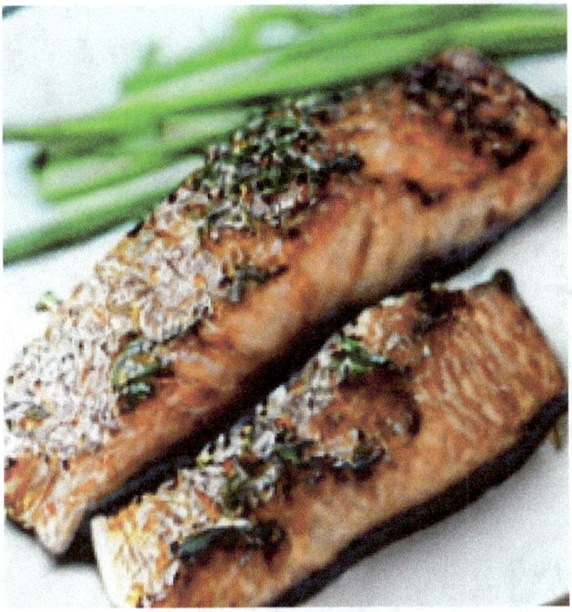

Ingredients:

- Salmon fillets
- Balsamic vinegar (low-sodium)
- Dijon mustard
- Honey
- Garlic, minced
- Olive oil
- Salt and pepper to taste

Preparation:

1. Whisk together balsamic vinegar, Dijon mustard, honey, minced garlic, olive oil, salt, and pepper to create a marinade.
2. Coat salmon fillets with the marinade and let them sit for a while.
3. Grill until the salmon is flaky and has a caramelized balsamic glaze.
4. This balsamic glazed grilled salmon is rich in omega-3 fatty acids and flavor.

Recipe 3. Mediterranean Vegetable Skewers

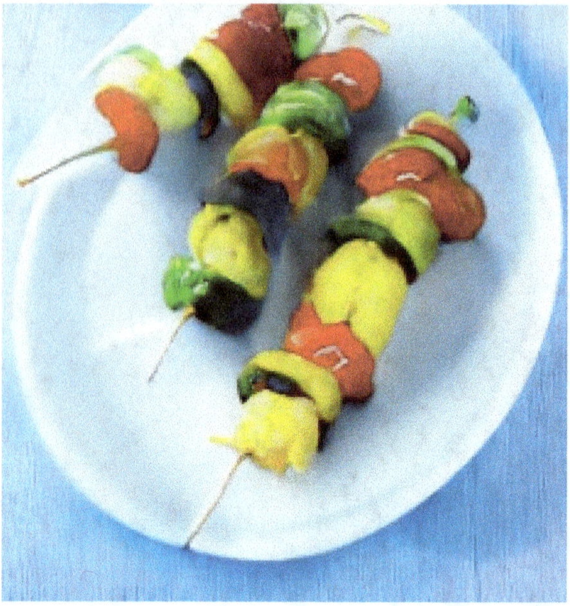

Ingredients:

- Cherry tomatoes
- Bell peppers, assorted colors, cut into chunks
- Zucchini, sliced
- Red onion, cut into wedges
- Olive oil
- Fresh oregano, chopped
- Lemon zest
- Salt and pepper to taste

Preparation:

1. Thread cherry tomatoes, bell peppers, zucchini, and red onion onto skewers.
2. Brush with olive oil, and sprinkle with chopped oregano, lemon zest, salt, and pepper.
3. Grill until veggies give under a gentle poke and show enticing grill marks.
4. These Mediterranean vegetable skewers offer a burst of colors and antioxidants.

Recipe 4. Teriyaki Tofu and Pineapple Kebabs

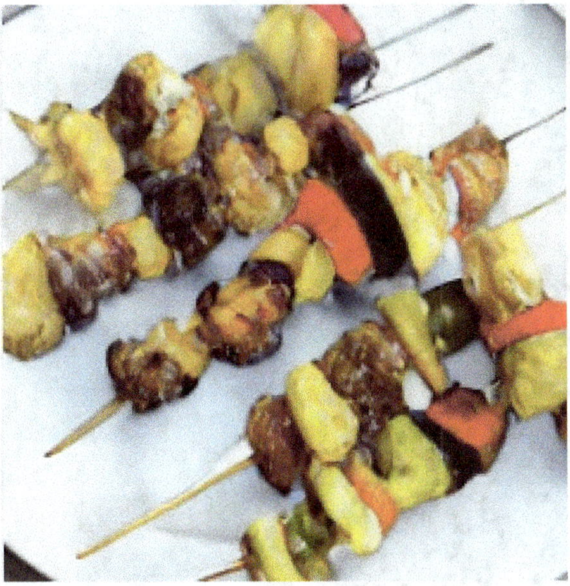

Ingredients:

- Extra-firm tofu, cubed
- Pineapple chunks
- Teriyaki sauce (low-sodium)
- Sesame oil
- Green onions, sliced
- Sesame seeds

Preparation:

1. Marinate tofu cubes and pineapple chunks in a mixture of low-sodium teriyaki sauce and sesame oil.
2. Thread them onto skewers, alternating between tofu and pineapple.
3. Grill until the kebabs have a golden glaze and are heated through.
4. Sprinkle with sliced green onions and sesame seeds for a flavorful tofu delight.

Recipe 5. Herb-Infused Grilled Eggplant

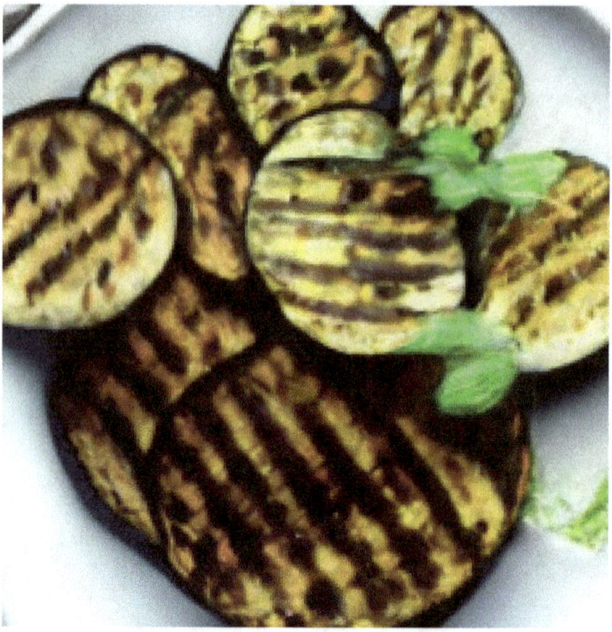

Ingredients:

- Eggplant, sliced
- Olive oil
- Fresh basil, chopped
- Fresh mint, chopped
- Garlic, minced
- Lemon juice
- Salt and pepper to taste

Preparation:

1. Brush eggplant slices with olive oil and sprinkle with chopped basil, mint, minced garlic, lemon juice, salt, and pepper.
2. Grill until the eggplant is tender and has a smoky essence.
3. This herb-infused grilled eggplant is a delicious and low-potassium option.

Recipe 6. Rosemary Garlic Grilled Shrimp Skewers

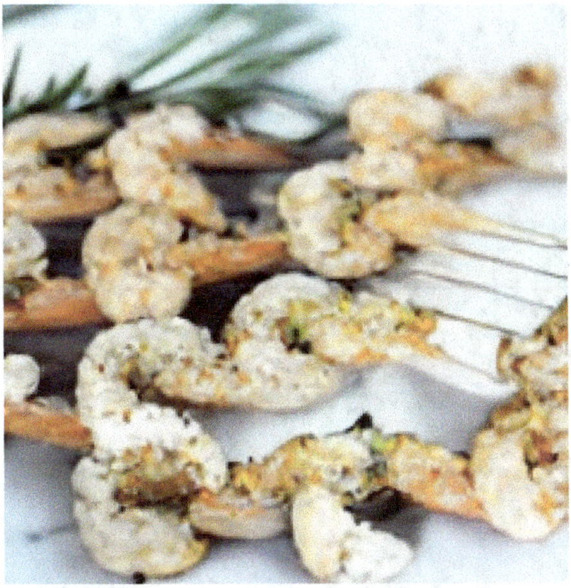

Ingredients:

- Shrimp, peeled and deveined
- Olive oil
- Fresh rosemary, chopped
- Garlic, minced
- Lemon zest
- Salt and pepper to taste

Preparation:

1. Toss shrimp with olive oil, chopped rosemary, minced garlic, lemon zest, salt, and pepper.
2. Thread them onto skewers.
3. Grill until the shrimp are opaque and infused with the aromatic flavors.
4. These rosemary garlic grilled shrimp skewers offer a delightful seafood option.

Recipe 7. Cumin-Spiced Grilled Vegetables

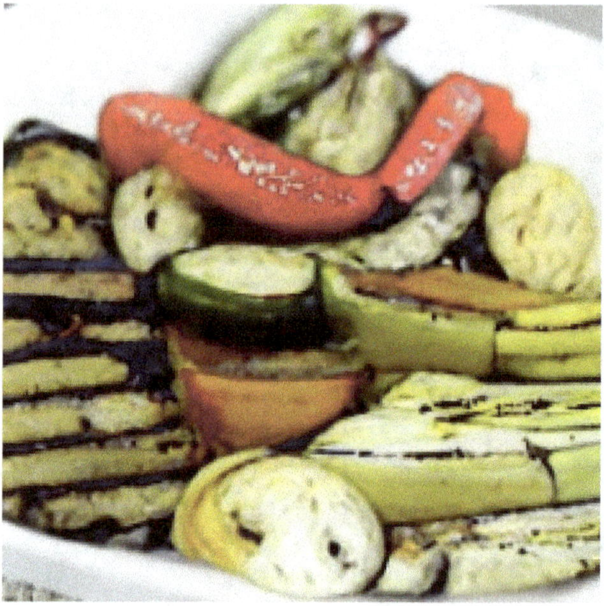

Ingredients:

- Cauliflower florets
- Broccoli florets
- Carrots, sliced
- Cumin powder
- Paprika
- Olive oil
- Fresh cilantro, chopped
- Lime wedges

Preparation:

1. Toss cauliflower, broccoli, and carrots with cumin powder, paprika, and olive oil.
2. Grill until the vegetables are lightly charred.
3. Garnish with cilantro and lime.
4. These cumin-spiced grilled vegetables provide a flavorful and kidney-friendly side dish.

Chapter 7
Snacks and Appetizers

Kidney-Friendly Snacking

Recipe 1. Roasted Chickpeas with Turmeric and Cumin

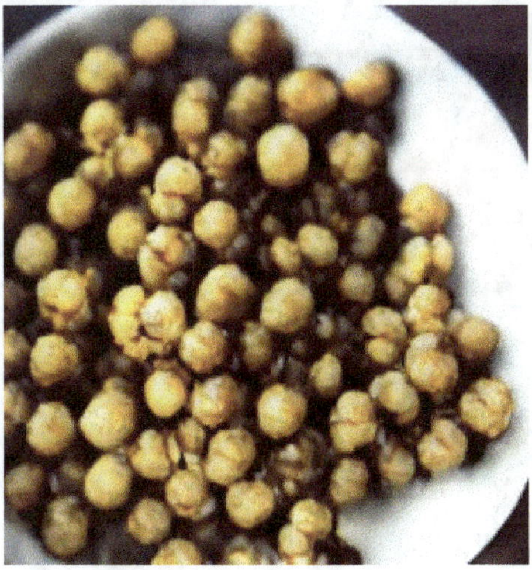

Ingredients:

- Canned chickpeas, drained and rinsed
- Olive oil
- Turmeric
- Cumin
- Garlic powder
- Salt and pepper to taste

Preparation:

1. Toss chickpeas with olive oil, turmeric, cumin, garlic powder, salt, and pepper.
2. Roast in the oven until golden and crunchy.
3. These roasted chickpeas are a protein-packed and spiced-up snack.

Recipe 2. Fresh Veggie Sticks with Hummus

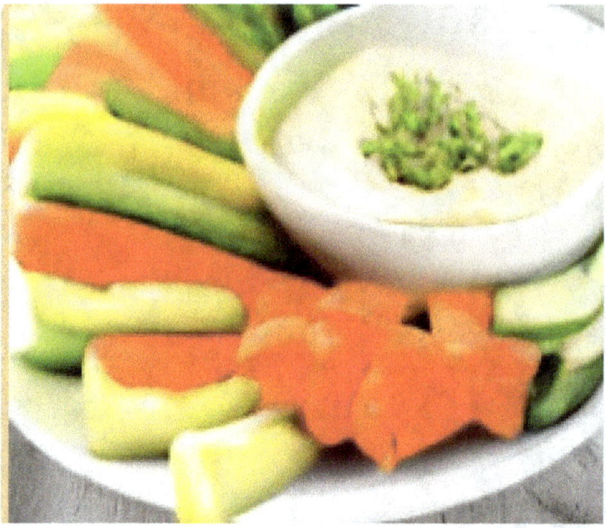

Ingredients:

- Carrot sticks
- Cucumber spears
- Bell pepper strips
- Cherry tomatoes
- Hummus (low-sodium)

Preparation:

1. Arrange carrot sticks, cucumber spears, bell pepper strips, and cherry tomatoes on a plate.
2. Pair with a side of low-sodium hummus for a refreshing and crunchy snack.
3. This veggie and hummus combo is a wholesome and hydrating option.

Recipe 3. Caprese Skewers with Balsamic Glaze

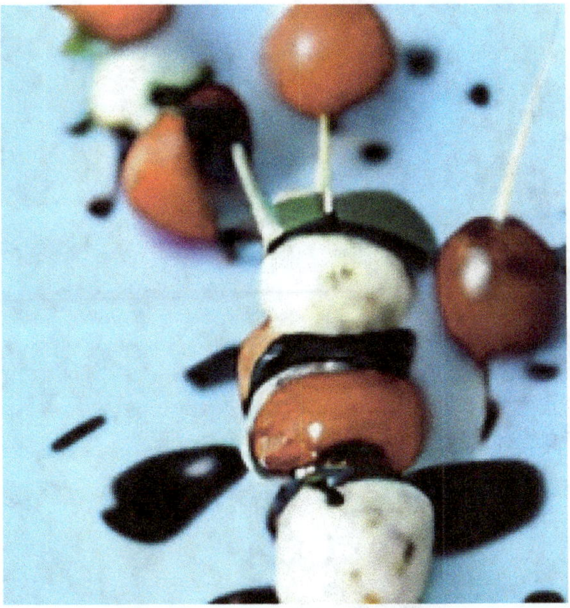

Ingredients:

- Cherry tomatoes
- Fresh mozzarella balls
- Basil leaves
- Balsamic glaze (low-sodium)

Preparation:

1. Assemble caprese skewers by alternating cherry tomatoes, mozzarella balls, and basil leaves.
2. Drizzle with low-sodium balsamic glaze.
3. These Caprese skewers offer a burst of freshness and Italian-inspired flavors.

Recipe 4. Greek Yogurt Parfait with Berries

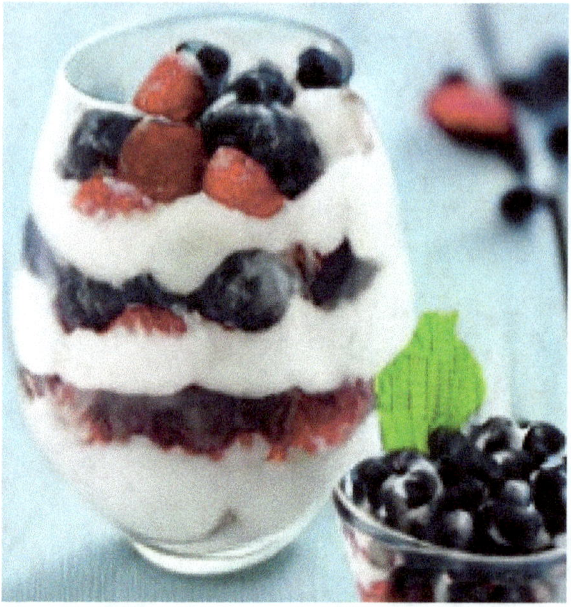

Ingredients:

- Greek yogurt
- Fresh berries (blueberries, strawberries, raspberries)
- Granola (low-phosphorus)

Preparation:

1. Layer Greek yogurt with fresh berries in a parfait glass.
2. Sprinkle with low-phosphorus granola for added crunch.
3. This Greek yogurt parfait is a protein-rich and satisfying sweet treat.

Recipe 5. Avocado and Tomato Salsa with Whole Grain Chips

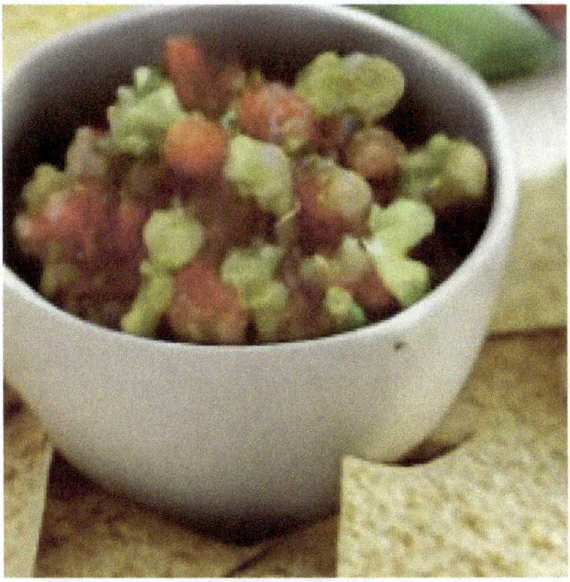

Ingredients:

- Avocado, diced
- Tomatoes, diced
- Red onion, finely chopped
- Fresh cilantro, chopped
- Lime juice
- Salt and pepper to taste
- Whole grain tortilla chips

Preparation:

1. Combine diced avocado, tomatoes, finely chopped red onion, and chopped cilantro.
2. Drizzle lime juice over the mixture and season it with salt and pepper.
3. Serve with whole-grain tortilla chips for a flavorful and heart-healthy dip.

Recipe 6. Cottage Cheese and Pineapple Boat

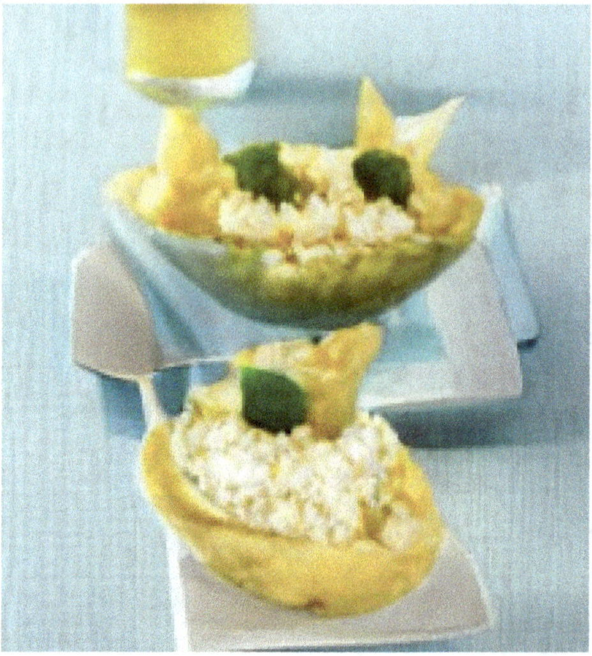

Ingredients:

- Cottage cheese
- Fresh pineapple, scooped into chunks
- Mint leaves, for garnish

Preparation:

1. Fill a hollowed-out pineapple half with cottage cheese.
2. Garnish with fresh mint leaves for a tropical and protein-packed snack.
3. This cottage cheese and pineapple boat is a refreshing and visually appealing treat.

Recipe 7. Almond Butter and Banana Slices

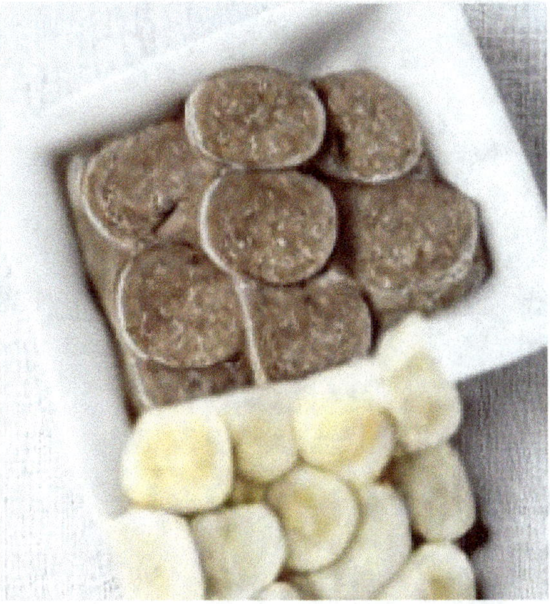

Ingredients:

- Banana, sliced
- Almond butter
- Chia seeds (optional)

Preparation:

1. Instructions:
2. Spread almond butter on banana slices.
3. Sprinkle with chia seeds for added texture if desired.
4. These almond butter and banana slices offer a combination of healthy fats and natural sweetness.

Recipe 8. Spinach and Feta Stuffed Mushrooms

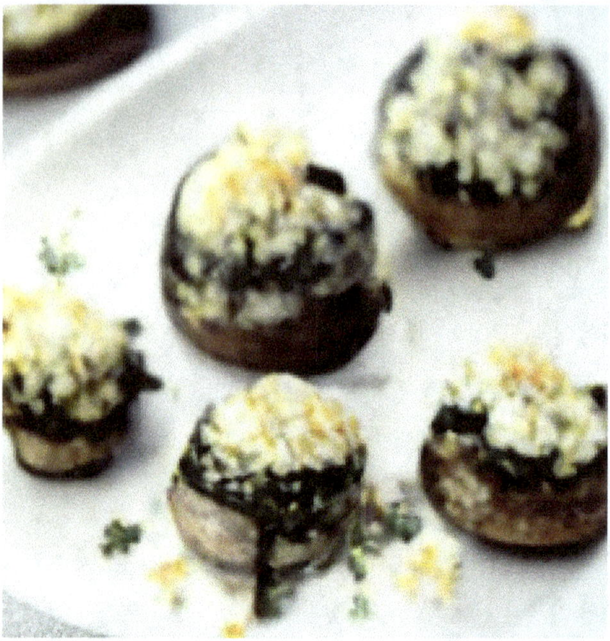

Ingredients:

- Mushrooms, cleaned and stems removed
- Frozen chopped spinach, thawed and drained
- Feta cheese, crumbled
- Garlic, minced
- Olive oil
- Black pepper to taste

Preparation:

1. Mix chopped spinach, crumbled feta, minced garlic, and a drizzle of olive oil.
2. Stuff mushrooms with the spinach and feta mixture.
3. Bake until the mushrooms soften and the filling reaches a golden glow.
4. These spinach and feta stuffed mushrooms are a savory and nutrient-rich appetizer.

Appetizers for Every Occasion

Recipe 1. Bruschetta Trio

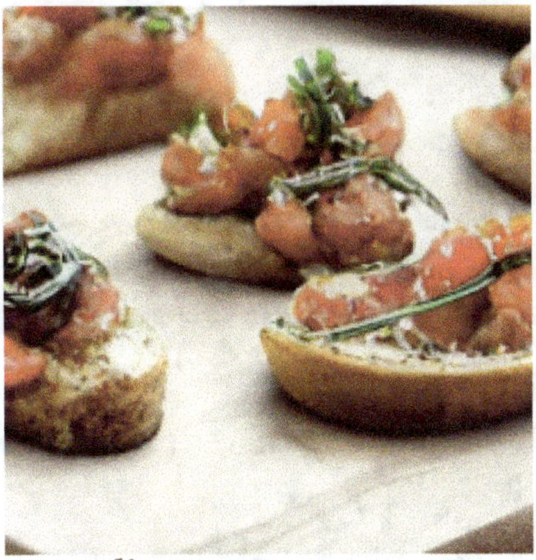

Preparation:

1. Toast baguette slices until golden.
2. Top each slice with a different bruschetta variation.
3. Arrange on a platter for a trio of flavors that cater to diverse palates.

Ingredients:

- Baguette slices
- Tomato and Basil Bruschetta:
- Diced tomatoes
- Fresh basil, chopped
- Garlic, minced
- Olive oil
- Balsamic glaze (optional)
- Avocado and Feta Bruschetta:
- Ripe avocado, mashed
- Feta cheese, crumbled
- Red pepper flakes
- Lemon zest
- Salt and pepper to taste
- Smoked Salmon and Cream Cheese Bruschetta:
- Smoked salmon
- Cream cheese
- Capers
- Fresh dill, chopped

Recipe 2. Stuffed Jalapeños with Bacon

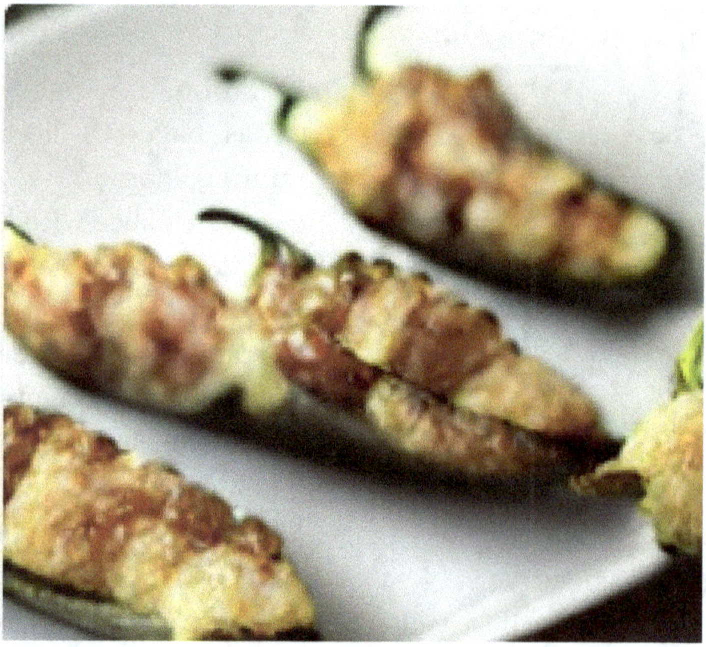

Ingredients:

- MuJalapeños, halved and seeded
- Cream cheese
- Cheddar cheese, shredded
- Green onions, chopped
- Bacon slices

Preparation:

1. Mix cream cheese, shredded cheddar, and chopped green onions.
2. Fill jalapeño halves with cream cheese mixture.
3. Wrap each jalapeño with a slice of bacon.
4. Grill until the bacon is crispy and the filling is melted.

Recipe 3. Spinach with Artichoke Dip with Pita Chips

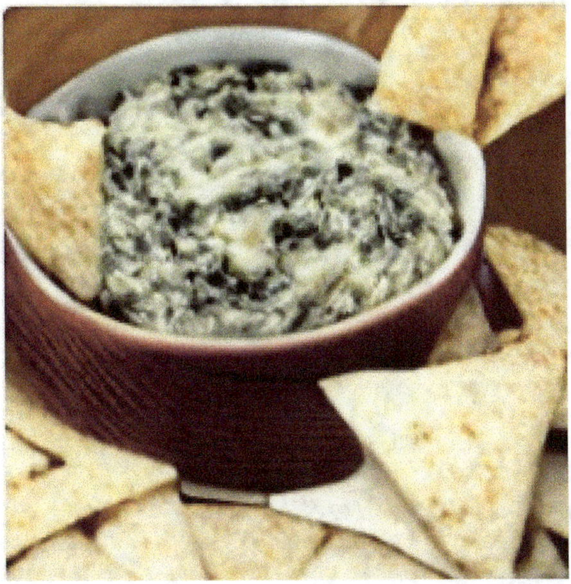

Ingredients:

- Frozen chopped spinach, thawed and drained
- Artichoke hearts, chopped
- Cream cheese
- Sour cream
- Parmesan cheese, grated
- Garlic, minced
- Pita chips for serving

Preparation:

1. Mix thawed spinach, chopped artichoke hearts, cream cheese, sour cream, grated Parmesan, and minced garlic.
2. Bake until the dip is bubbly and golden.
3. Serve with crispy pita chips for a crowd-pleasing appetizer.

Recipe 4. Mango Shrimp Ceviche

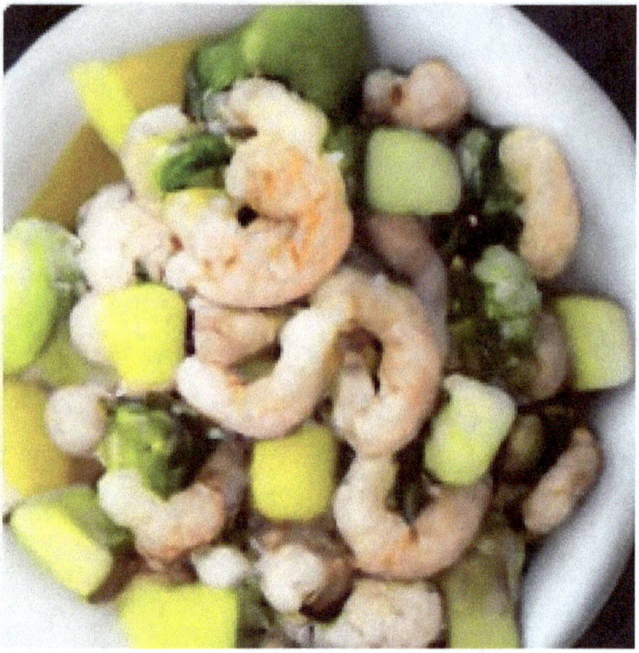

Ingredients:

- Shrimp, cooked and chopped
- Mango, diced
- Red onion, finely chopped
- Cilantro, chopped
- Lime juice
- Jalapeño, finely chopped
- Salt and pepper to taste
- Tortilla chips for serving

Preparation:

1. Combine cooked shrimp, diced mango, chopped red onion, chopped cilantro, lime juice, and chopped jalapeño.
2. Season with salt and pepper.
3. Chill before serving with tortilla chips for a refreshing ceviche.

Recipe 5. Mini Caprese Skewers

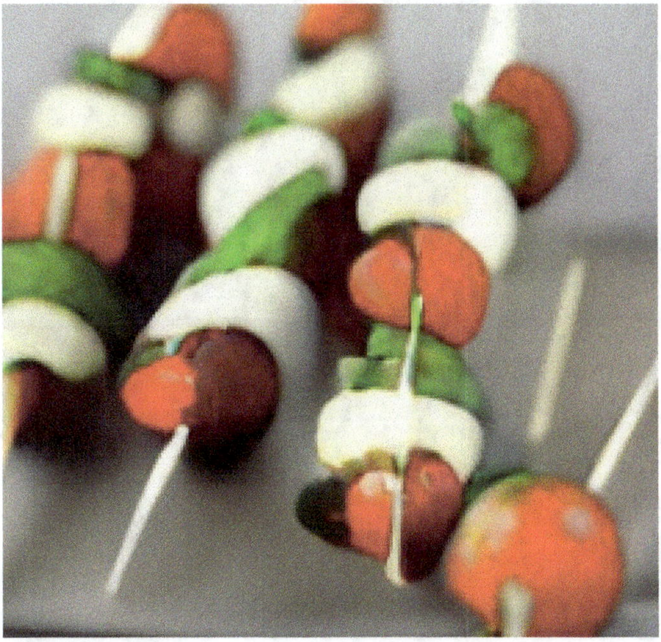

Ingredients:

- Cherry tomatoes
- Fresh mozzarella balls
- Basil leaves
- Balsamic glaze (optional)
- Toothpicks

Preparation:

1. Create bite-sized appetizers by threading cherry tomatoes, mozzarella balls, and basil leaves onto toothpicks.
2. Arrange on a platter and drizzle with balsamic glaze if desired.
3. These mini caprese skewers are a bite-sized burst of Italian flavors.

Recipe 6. Teriyaki Chicken Lettuce Wraps

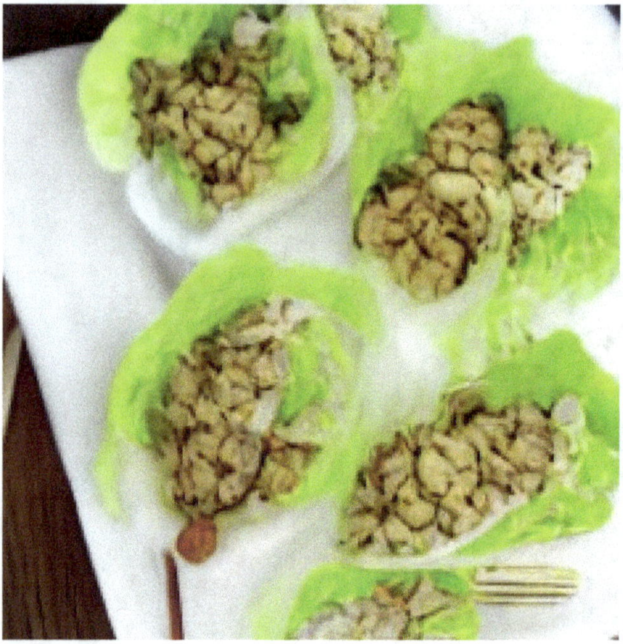

Ingredients:

- Grilled chicken, shredded
- Teriyaki sauce (low-sodium)
- Lettuce leaves
- Carrots, julienned
- Cucumber, julienned
- Green onions, sliced
- Sesame seeds for garnish

Preparation:

1. Toss shredded chicken in low-sodium teriyaki sauce.
2. Spoon the chicken into lettuce leaves.
3. Top with julienned carrots, cucumber, and sliced green onions.
4. Sprinkle with sesame seeds for an Asian-inspired appetizer.

Recipe 7. Mediterranean Hummus Platter

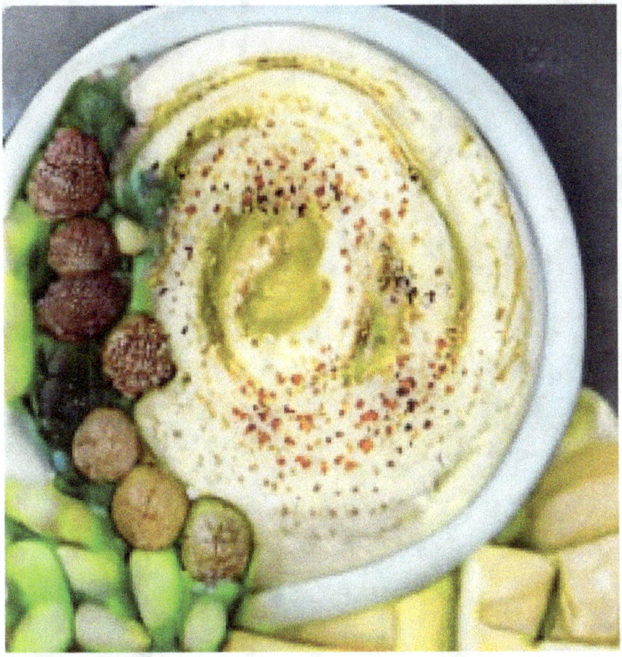

Ingredients:

- Hummus
- Cherry tomatoes
- Cucumber, sliced
- Kalamata olives
- Feta cheese, crumbled
- Pita bread, cut into wedges

Preparation:

1. Spread hummus on a serving platter.
2. Arrange cherry tomatoes, cucumber slices, Kalamata olives, and crumbled feta on top.
3. Serve with pita bread wedges for a Mediterranean-inspired delight.

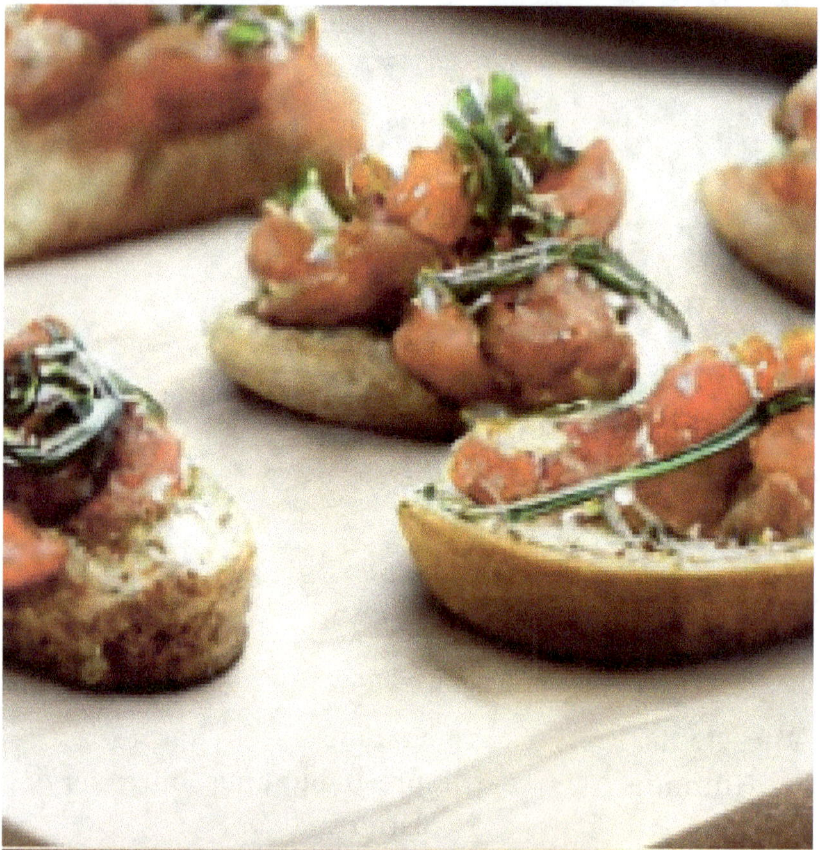

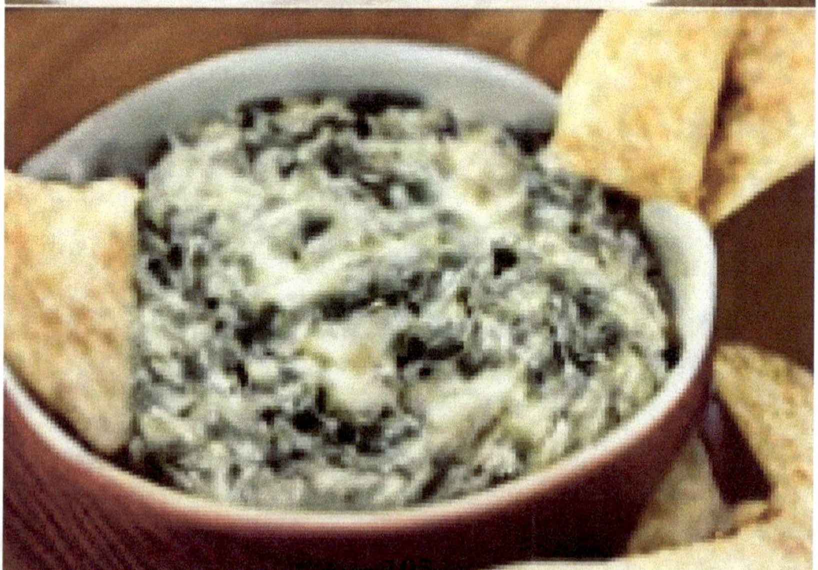

Chapter 8
Desserts with Care

Sweet Treats for Kidney-Friendly Diets

Recipe 1. Berry Parfait with Almond Crumble

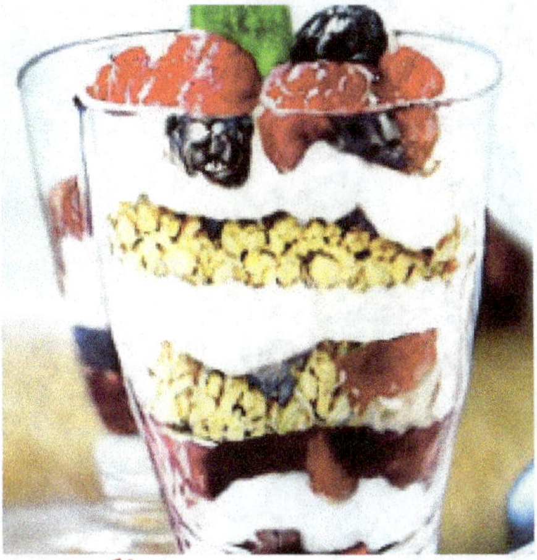

Ingredients:

- Mixed berries (strawberries, blueberries, raspberries)
- Greek yogurt
- Almonds, crushed
- Honey (optional)

Preparation:

1. Layer mixed berries with Greek yogurt in serving glasses.
2. In a separate bowl, mix crushed almonds with honey (if using).
3. Sprinkle the almond crumble over the berry and yogurt layers.
4. Repeat the layers and finish with a dollop of Greek yogurt on top.
5. This berry parfait with almond crumble is a refreshing and protein-packed dessert.

Recipe 2. Avocado Chocolate Mousse

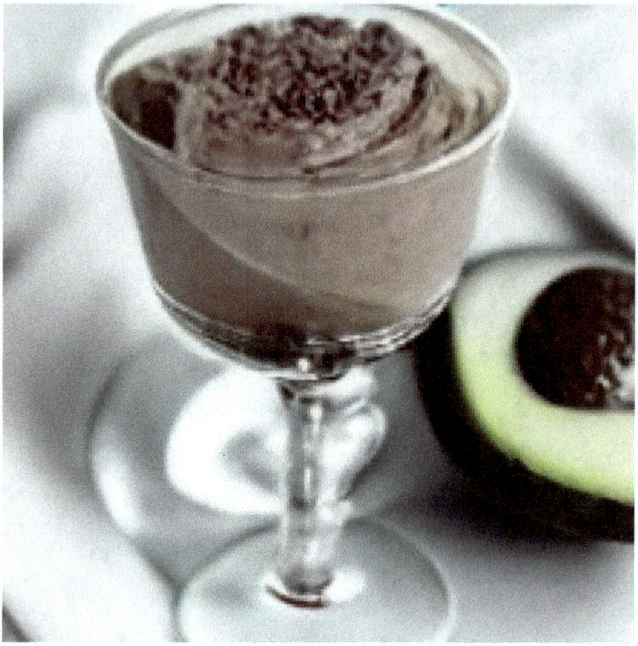

Ingredients:

- Ripe avocados, peeled and pitted
- Unsweetened cocoa powder
- Maple syrup or honey
- Vanilla extract
- Almond milk (unsweetened)
- Fresh berries for garnish

Preparation:

1. In a blender, combine ripe avocados, cocoa powder, maple syrup or honey, and vanilla extract.
2. Gradually add almond milk until the mixture is smooth and creamy.
3. Chill the chocolate mousse in the refrigerator.
4. Serve topped with fresh berries for a decadent yet kidney-friendly dessert.

Recipe 3. Chia Seed Pudding with Mango Puree

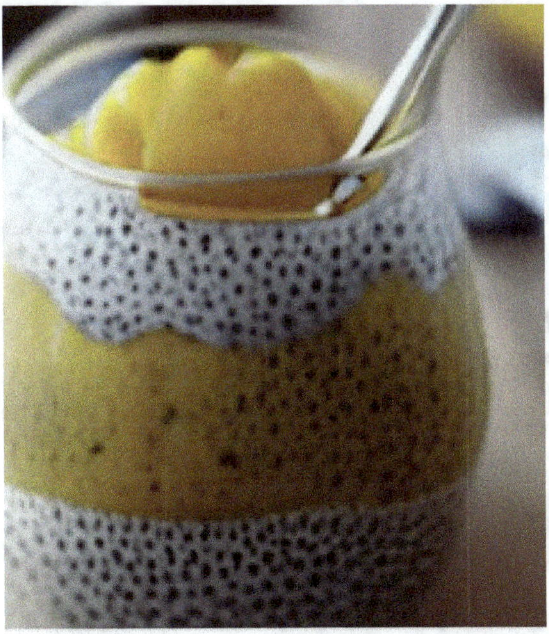

Ingredients:

- Ripe avocados, peeled and pitted
- Unsweetened cocoa powder
- Maple syrup or honey
- Vanilla extract
- Almond milk (unsweetened)
- Fresh berries for garnish

Preparation:

1. In a blender, combine ripe avocados, cocoa powder, maple syrup or honey, and vanilla extract.
2. Gradually add almond milk until the mixture is smooth and creamy.
3. Chill the chocolate mousse in the refrigerator.
4. Serve topped with fresh berries for a decadent yet kidney-friendly dessert.

Indulgent Desserts without Compromising Health

Recipe 1. Dark Chocolate Avocado Mousse

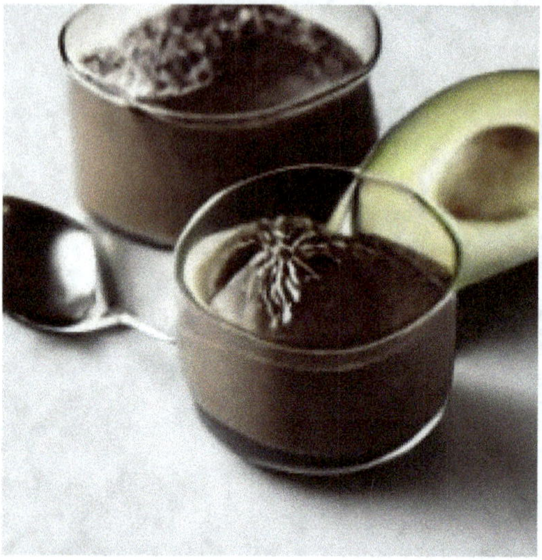

Ingredients:

- Ripe avocados, peeled and pitted
- Dark chocolate melted (70% cocoa or higher)
- Maple syrup or agave nectar
- Vanilla extract
- Pinch of sea salt
- Fresh berries for garnish

Preparation:

1. In a blender, combine ripe avocados, melted dark chocolate, maple syrup or agave nectar, vanilla extract, and a pinch of sea salt.
2. Blend until smooth and creamy.
3. Chill the mousse in the refrigerator.
4. Serve in individual bowls or glasses, garnished with fresh berries.
5. This dark chocolate avocado mousse is a luscious and health-conscious dessert.

Recipe 2. Nutty Banana Ice Cream

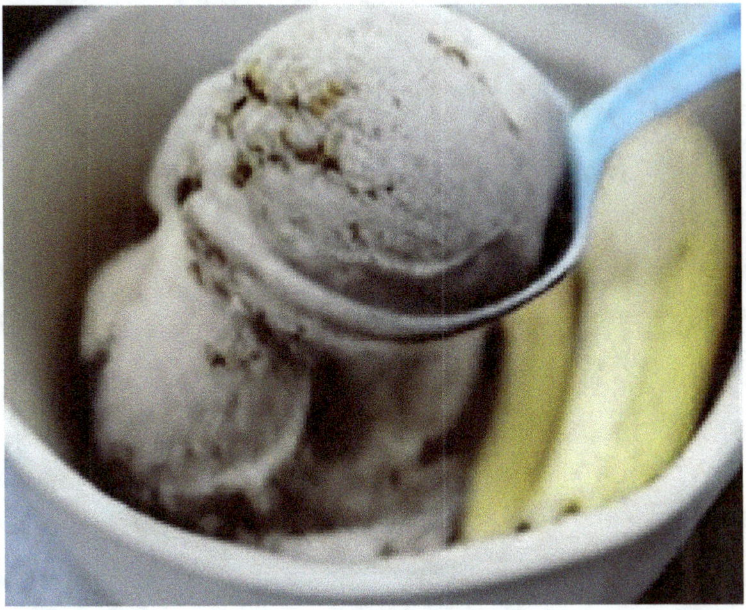

Ingredients:

- Ripe bananas, sliced and frozen
- Almond butter or peanut butter
- Almond milk (unsweetened)
- Chopped nuts for topping

Preparation:

1. In a food processor, blend frozen banana slices, almond butter or peanut butter, and a splash of unsweetened almond milk.
2. Blend until the mixture has a smooth and creamy consistency.
3. Scoop the banana ice cream into bowls.
4. Top with chopped nuts for added crunch.
5. This nutty banana ice cream is a delightful and wholesome frozen treat.

Recipe 3. Baked Apples with Cinnamon and Walnuts

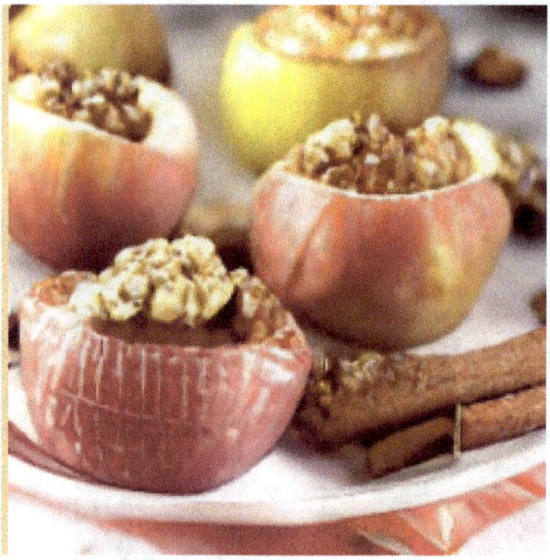

Ingredients:

- Apples, cored and halved
- Ground cinnamon
- Chopped walnuts
- Honey or maple syrup
- Greek yogurt for serving

Preparation:

1. Preheat the oven to 375°F (190°C).
2. Place cored and halved apples on a baking sheet.
3. Sprinkle with ground cinnamon and chopped walnuts.
4. Drizzle with honey or maple syrup.
5. Bake until the apples becomes tender and shows a golden color.
6. Serve with a dollop of Greek yogurt for a warm and comforting dessert.

Chapter 9
Beverages for Kidney Health

Recipe 1. Citrus Infused Water: Summer Freshness

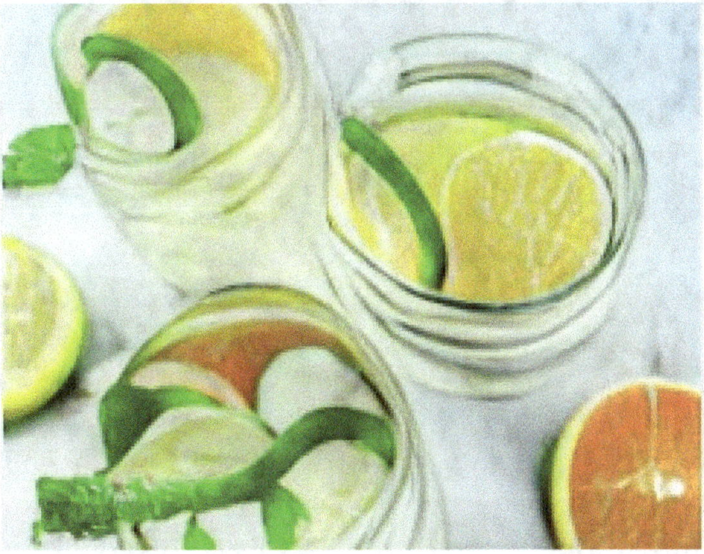

Ingredients:

- Lemon slices
- Lime slices
- Orange slices
- Fresh mint leaves
- Ice cubes
- Water

Preparation:

1. Add lemons, limes, and oranges to a pitcher
2. Add fresh mint leaves and ice cubes.
3. Fill the pitcher with water and refrigerate.
4. This citrus-infused water is a hydrating and invigorating drink for hot summer days

Recipe 2. Hibiscus Iced Tea: Autumn Bliss

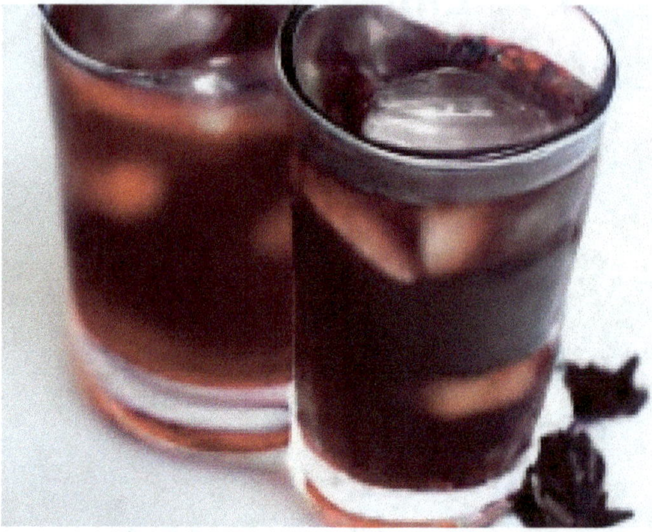

Ingredients:

- Hibiscus tea bags
- Boiling water
- Orange peel
- Cinnamon stick
- Honey or agave syrup (optional)
- Ice cubes

Preparation:

1. Steep hibiscus tea bags in boiling water.
2. Add orange peel and a cinnamon stick to infuse flavor.
3. For sweetness, add honey or agave syrup to taste.
4. Chill and serve over ice.
5. This hibiscus iced tea is a fragrant and kidney-friendly autumn beverage.

Recipe 3. Warm Ginger Turmeric Milk: Winter Comfort

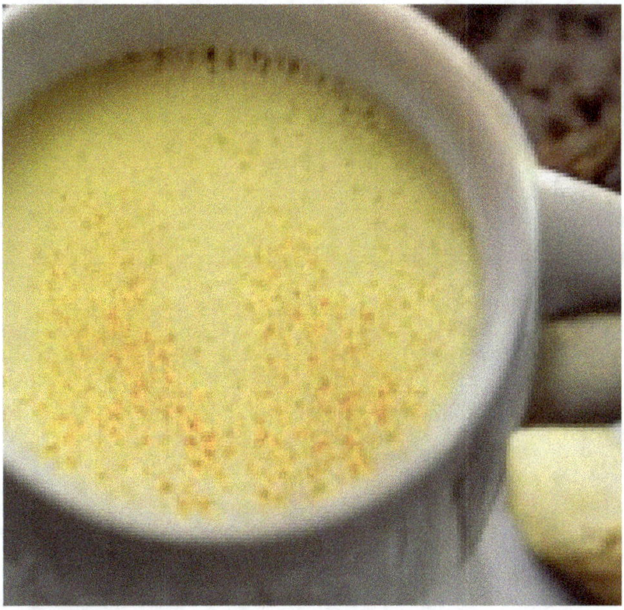

Ingredients:

- Almond milk (unsweetened)
- Ground ginger
- Ground turmeric
- Honey or maple syrup
- Ground cinnamon (optional)

Preparation:

1. Heat almond milk in a saucepan.
2. Stir in ground ginger and ground turmeric.
3. Add honey or maple syrup for sweetness to taste.
4. Add a sprinkle of ground cinnamon if desired.
5. This warm ginger turmeric milk provides comfort and immune support during the winter months.

Recipe 4. Green Tea with Mint and Cucumber: Spring Revitalization

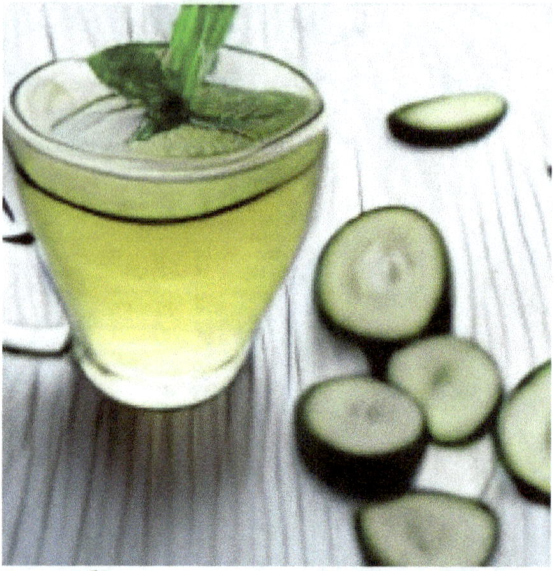

Ingredients:

- Green tea bags
- Boiling water
- Fresh mint leaves
- Cucumber slices
- Lemon wedges
- Ice cubes

Preparation:

1. Steep green tea bags in boiling water.
2. Add fresh mint leaves and cucumber slices.
3. Allow the tea to cool, then refrigerate.
4. Serve over ice with lemon wedges.
5. This green tea with mint and cucumber offers a refreshing and revitalizing sip for spring.

Chapter 10
Meal Planning and Preparation
Building a Kidney-Friendly Meal Plan

In this chapter, we delve into the art of crafting a kidney-friendly meal plan and the essential tips for successful meal preparation. Building a nourishing diet tailored to support kidney health requires thoughtful planning and efficient preparation. Let's explore the key principles behind creating a well-balanced meal plan and the strategies to streamline the process of preparing wholesome, kidney-friendly meals.

1. Balance Macronutrients:

- Incorporate a balance of macronutrients, including protein, carbohydrates, and healthy fats.
- Opt for lean protein sources such as poultry, fish, tofu, and legumes to manage protein intake effectively.
- Choose complex carbohydrates like whole grains, fruits, and vegetables to provide sustained energy.

2. Monitor Phosphorus and Potassium:

- Keep an eye on phosphorus and potassium levels, as imbalances can impact kidney function.
- Limit high-phosphorus foods such as dairy products, nuts, and processed foods.
- Choose low-potassium options like berries, apples, and cauliflower to maintain electrolyte balance.

3. Control Sodium Intake:

- Manage sodium intake to help regulate blood pressure and fluid balance.
- Opt for fresh, whole foods and limit the use of processed and packaged items.
- Experiment with herbs and spices for flavor without relying heavily on salt.

4. Include Kidney-Friendly Superfoods:

- Incorporate superfoods known for their kidney-friendly properties, such as blueberries, cabbage, and cauliflower.
- Explore nutrient-dense options like kale, bell peppers, and onions to enhance the nutritional profile of your meals.

5. Hydration is Key:

- Stay well-hydrated by including beverages like water, herbal teas, and infused water in your daily routine.
- Limit the consumption of sugary drinks and caffeinated beverages, and consult with your healthcare provider to determine the optimal fluid intake for your condition.

Tips for Successful Meal Preparation

1. Batch Cooking:

- Prepare ingredients in larger quantities to create multiple meals at once.
- Portion and store meals in the refrigerator or freezer for convenient and quick access during busy days.

2. Pre-Cut and Pre-Wash:

- Wash and chop fruits, vegetables, and herbs in advance to save time during meal preparation.
- Store pre-cut items in sealed containers to maintain freshness.

3. Create a Weekly Menu:

- Plan your meals for the week, considering variety and nutritional balance.
- Create a shopping list based on your menu to streamline grocery shopping.

4. Utilize Slow Cookers and Instant Pots:

- Embrace the convenience of slow cookers and Instant Pots for hands-free cooking.
- These appliances are excellent for preparing stews, soups, and one-pot meals with minimal effort.

5. Label and Date:

- Label and date containers to track the freshness of prepared meals.
- Ensure that perishable items are consumed within a safe timeframe.

6. ***Experiment with Flavors:***

- Explore different herbs, spices, and low-sodium seasonings to add variety and excitement to your meals.
- Experimenting with flavors can make kidney-friendly dishes more enjoyable.

7. ***Consult with a Dietitian:***

- Seek guidance from a registered dietitian to personalize your meal plan based on your specific dietary needs and restrictions.
- Regular consultations can help fine-tune your approach to kidney-friendly nutrition.

By incorporating these principles into your meal planning and preparation routine, you can create a sustainable and kidney-friendly approach to eating. Nourish your body with care, and enjoy the benefits of wholesome, flavorful meals that support your overall well-being.

Conclusion

As we conclude this journey through "Comfort Foods for Chronic Kidney Disease: Nourishing, Kidney-Friendly Recipes to Enjoy While Managing Dialysis, Minerals, and Nutrition," it is our hope that this guide has served as a valuable companion on your path to kidney-friendly living.

In these pages, we've explored the intricacies of managing dialysis, understanding essential minerals for kidney health, and crafting nutrient-packed recipes that not only support your well-being but also tantalize your taste buds. From comforting breakfasts to satisfying lunches, indulgent desserts, and refreshing beverages, each chapter has been meticulously designed to empower you with the knowledge and tools needed to embrace a nourishing lifestyle.

The heart of this book lies in the recognition that managing Chronic Kidney Disease requires more than just dietary adjustments, it calls for a holistic approach to health. Through carefully curated recipes, insightful information, and practical tips on meal planning and preparation, we've aimed to provide you with a comprehensive resource that fosters well-being in every aspect of your life.

Remember, the journey to kidney-friendly living is unique to each individual. It is a journey marked by resilience, self-discovery, and a commitment to making choices that prioritize your health and happiness.

As you embark on this path, we encourage you to engage with your healthcare team, explore the delicious recipes offered in this book, and find joy in the process of nourishing both your body and your soul.

May these pages continue to inspire you on your quest for comfort, flavor, and kidney-friendly vitality. From our kitchen to yours, here's to a life filled with delicious moments and well-nourished joy. Embrace the comfort foods that care for your kidneys, savor the flavors that bring warmth to your heart, and relish in the richness of a life well-lived with chronic kidney disease.

www.ingramcontent.com/pod-product-compliance
Lightning Source LLC
Chambersburg PA
CBHW070853260726
48661CB00004B/1390
* 9 7 9 8 8 7 4 4 8 1 9 3 3 *